S0-ERB-255

WITHDRAWN

WILLIAM F. MAAG LIBRARY
YOUNGSTOWN STATE UNIVERSITY

PLASMA PROTEIN PATHOLOGY

PLASMA PROTEIN PATHOLOGY

A workshop on plasma proteins, their availability, assay and therapeutic uses

Edited by

HUBERT PEETERS

Lipid & Protein Dept, LBS, Brussels, Belgium

and

PETER H. WRIGHT

Travenol International
Brussels, Belgium

PERGAMON PRESS

OXFORD · NEW YORK · TORONTO · SYDNEY · PARIS · FRANKFURT

U.K.	Pergamon Press Ltd., Headington Hill Hall, Oxford OX3 0BW, England
U.S.A.	Pergamon Press Inc., Maxwell House, Fairview Park, Elmsford, New York 10523, U.S.A.
CANADA	Pergamon of Canada Ltd., 75 The East Mall, Toronto, Ontario, Canada
AUSTRALIA	Pergamon Press (Aust.) Pty. Ltd., P.O. Box 544, Potts Point, N.S.W. 2011, Australia
FRANCE	Pergamon Press SARL, 24 rue des Ecoles, 75240 Paris, Cedex 05, France
FEDERAL REPUBLIC OF GERMANY	Pergamon Press GmbH, 6242 Kronberg-Taunus, Pferdstrasse 1, Federal Republic of Germany

---

Copyright © 1979 Pergamon Press Ltd.

All Rights Reserved. No part of this publication may be reproduced, stored in a retrieval system or transmitted in any form or by any means: electronic, electrostatic, magnetic tape, mechanical, photocopying, recording or otherwise, without permission in writing from the publishers.

First edition 1979

British Library Cataloguing in Publication Data

Plasma protein pathology.
1. Blood proteins - Congresses
I. Peeters, Hubert II. Wright, Peter H
612'12 QP99.3.P7 78-40994

ISBN 0-08-023766-5

In order to make this volume available as economically and as rapidly as possible the authors' typescripts have been reproduced in their original forms. This method unfortunately has its typographical limitations but it is hoped that they in no way distract the reader.

Printed and bound at William Clowes & Sons Limited Beccles and London

QP
99.3
.P7P56
1979

Contents

WILLIAM F. MAAG LIBRARY
YOUNGSTOWN STATE UNIVERSITY

Participants

Professor Rudy E. Ballieux
Akademisch Ziekenhuis Utrecht
Immunologisch Laboratorium
Katarijnensingel, 101
NL - Utrecht, Holland

Dr. Gregory J. Buffone
Children's Hospital
National Medical Center
111 Michigan Avenue
Washington, DC20010, USA

Dr. Ralph E. Dolkart
Travenol International Services, Inc.
Chaussée de la Hulpe, 130
1050 - Brussels, Belgium

Professor Robert Engler
Université René Descartes
UER Biomédicale des Saints Pères
Département de Biochimie
45 rue des Saints Pères
75070 - Paris Cedex 010, France

Professor John R. Hobbs
Protein Reference Unit
Westminster Medical School
London, W.1., England

Professor Dr. Hans W. Intorp
Medizinische Univ.-Poliklinik
Westring 3
D 4400 Münster/Germany

Mr. Herwig Leyssens
S.A. Travenol N.V.
Boulevard d'Houraing
7860 Lessines, Belgium

Professor Pierre L. Masson
Unité de Médecine Expérimentale
Université Catholique de Louvain
Avenue Hippocrate, 75
1200, Brussels, Belgium

Dr. Christian Mathot
International Technical Services
Hyland Products Division
3300 Hyland Avenue
Costa Mesa, California 92626 U.S.A.

Dr. Hubert Peeters
Lipid And Protein Department, LBS
196 Alsembergsesteenweg
B-1180 Brussels, Belgium

Professor Jose Luis Serrera
Laboratorio Bioquimica Clinica
Residencia "Garcia Morato"
Ciudad Sanitaria "Virgen del Rocio"
Avenida Manuel Siurot
Sevilla, Spain

Dr. Peter H. Wright
Travenol International Services, Inc.
Chaussée de la Hulpe, 130
1050- Brussels
Belgium

Dr. René De Vreker
Hyland Division
Travenol Laboratories, Inc.
3300 Hyland Avenue
Costa Mesa, California 92626
U.S.A.

Introduction

Ralph E. Dolkart

Brussels, Belgium

This workshop was sponsored by Travenol International Services, Hyland Division, Brussels, Belgium. Although many large national and international meetings have dealt with various aspects of the topics presented here, it was felt that by bringing together a small group of experts in an informal setting an easier and more profitable exchange of ideas would be possible.

The topics of this workshop reflect the development of medical knowledge since the turn of the century.From the late 19th century until the mid-1920's interest was focused on correlation of clinical findings and the autopsy table. Next until about 1935 a pharmacologic era when responses of tissues and organs to various drugs were of primary concern. Then came a physiological and biochemical eras followed, by a period (1945) in which there was rapid development in cellular and molecular biology. At this time, and stimulated by advances made during World War II, development of sophisticated laboratory methods heralded an immunological era. Fractionation of plasma became possible and by the study of plasma protein components certain disease states became more readily identifiable. Administration of blood protein fractions proved either curative or, at the least, life sustaining. Removal of abnormal proteins or of other constituents of blood by plasmapheresis resulted in amelioration of some disease states. New concepts of therapy emerged. Against this background this meeting was held.

Travenol is grateful for the efforts of the participants; for the diligence shown by Dr.Hubert Peeters and Dr. Peter Wright who edited this volume; for the skill and patience of Mme Isabelle Ragheb who typed and corrected the manuscripts; and for the arrangements made for the meeting by Mr.John Hart and Sra Nina Miralles of the Travenol offices in Brussels and Valencia. Finally, I would like, on behalf of all participants, to thank Professor Serrera and his wife who were our hosts during this short but very pleasant visit to Seville, Spain.

Therapeutic Potentials of Plasma Proteins

Hubert Peeters

Brussels, Belgium

This workshop will cover a set of papers and discussions centered around two connected topics, Therapeutic needs and Assay methods for individual plasma proteins. Each participant has a different background in the protein field and so the focus of interest will shift around such questions as the levels of several specific plasma proteins, the availability of specific proteins and the rationale for their replacement. It looks as if discussions should have been rescheduled according to the following sequence. First, determination of protein levels should have been considered, then the rationale for their replacement and finally their availability. This logic did not prevail because our main objective was to generate new insights, to broaden our outlook, to compare points of view and to generate some imaginative thinking around plasma proteins. For this reason discussion of assay methods, the more straight forward topic, was left to the last, while the natural history of plasma proteins came first and problems of replacement of depleted fractions second. Let us start with an introductory subjective overview of the potential of this workshop.

PROBLEMS ASSOCIATED WITH SPECIFIC THERAPEUTIC REQUIREMENTS

The need for whole plasma as a plasma substitute is not "dépassé" - it never shall be - but the replacement of individual proteins has become increasingly important. As the needs for individual proteins increase, so grow the problems of supply. Can we envisage new sources of supply ? At first sight there is an unsurmountable immunological barrier prohibiting use of non-human protein. If tissue proteins are considered, this problem becomes even more difficult, if not impossible, to surmount. This immunological barrier could be avoided either if the recipient were made indifferent to the foreign protein or if the replacement material itself were indifferent. The first mechanism, involving the patient, is being approached by physical and chemical means. Unfortunately, however, there are no specific inhibitors available which protect the patient against reactions to one antigen while maintaining his defense machanism alert to deal with other truly offending agents. A century ago, Besredka introduced a simple trick to circumvent the immunological response against anti-tetanus serum, and it is still in use. To the best of my knowledge, little else has been developed since then. Another approach to substitution therapy would be the preparation of neutral proteins. The term "neutral" might be better than "immunologically inactive", not only because it is shorter, but also because it does not imply that the molecule has absolutely no antigenic potential.

What is the status of affairs regarding (a) sequences of amino acids having biological activity but low or negligible antigenicity; and (b) compounds which could from the immunological point of view cover up the immunogenically active sequence of a polypeptide without destroying therapeutic function.

On the first point, the amino acids of many proteins with biological activity have been sequenced and the comparative anatomy of their chemical backbone is interesting. From the apopolypeptides (i.e. the delipidated polypeptides of lipoproteins) one learns that only segments of the molecule carry the lipid and for this reason relatively short synthetic polypeptides could be designed to perform this task. What about their antigenicity ? Could we have a sequence capable of removing lipid physiologically but having no specific immunogenicity within the human species? Indeed, it appears that some polypeptide hormones, as well as the apopolypeptides of our lipoproteins, are common to many species with practically the same sequence in all. Could we then extract specific lipid binding polypeptides from animal serum? Should we synthesize the correct sequence? Could we select animals, plants, bacteria or even viruses to perform polypeptide production as we have done for other active substances? Genetic engineering could be important with such a goal in mind. The second hypothesis would require introduction of polypeptides or proteins covered by a chemical which can mask antigenic sites without destroying therapeutic potential. Can we devise ligands adapted to the job ? To my knowledge the differences observed between sera raised against an apoprotein or its lipid loaded counterpart provide a useful hint in this direction.

From a general point of view, therapy by replacement of proteins can be subdivided into three categories. First, there are proteins acting on a bulk basis, as is true for albumin, gammaglobulins, etc. Secondly they may act as transport proteins, e.g. lipid removal through apoproteins as proposed above. Lastly, there are those which act in trace amounts e.g. hormones, blood clotting enzymes, complement factors, etc. The diagnostic use of some proteins or polypeptides must also be mentioned in this context. In conclusion, applicability of proteins to a practical therapeutic goal is basically linked to the immunological problem but has to be preceded by a careful evaluation of needs. This implies rapid measurements of the deficient level and/or of excessive metabolic turnover and follow-up of pre-and post therapy levels to be discussed later under the heading of protein assay. We could also attempt to establish a list of the accepted and treatable deficiencies as well as potential ones for which protein fractions should be selected for preparative efforts in the future. This gremium could make useful suggestions in this respect.

AVAILABILITY OF PROTEINS TO COVER THERAPEUTIC REQUIREMENTS

Many of us are associated with production of liquid and frozen human plasma. There has been a Spanish attempt to produce heated bovine plasma derivatives as non-antigenic human plasma substitutes but it was unsuccessful. Later, in this same peninsula, at Lisbon, Kohn demonstrated chemical precipitation of plasma proteins in a continuous centrifugal separator of his own design. Later developments, heralded by Tiselius and based on monospecific affinity columns, yielded far more homogenous individual fractions. We are now near to the ultimate goal of purity in the manufacture of specific clotting factors and gammaglobulins.

One of the ideas I would like to rekindle is that of an anticoagulant with promising aspects. Instead of sodium citrate one could use sodium lactate as a calcium ligand. The peculiar property of this chemical is its non-removable hydration water. This means that sodium lactate is never available as a salt but only as a concentrated solution. As a result plasma or protein concentrates can be obtained as pastes, not as powders, a process requiring less effort than complete lyophilysation. To our knowledge the potential of this idea has not yet been tried out. It is interesting to remember that lactate accumulating in muscle is responsible for pain and stiffness after muscular exertion. This pain could result from water retention and swelling of muscle cells and might not be solely due to decrease in pH. We have used sodium lactate as an anticoagulant in thousands of transfusions over the years and believe it to be a practical and interesting calcium chelator and anticoagulant.

EDTA acts as an excellent calcium buffer, thus reducing enzyme activity. For this reason it is the preferred anticoagulant in analysis of plasma lipoproteins. This could mean that plasma for production of a specific protein should be drawn into an anti-coagulant specifically chosen to improve the quality and yield of the final material.

Another problem occurs in plasma protein production using ion-exchange columns exposed to large amounts of non-fasting plasma. Such plasma often contains chylomicra and VLDL (Very Low Density Lipoproteins), which are all too ready to shed part of their lipid and clog the column at low temperature. Partial Freon delipidation by removal of triglycerides is useful in this respect and is already being applied in this context for the preparation of improved reference sera for the WHO. Could this idea be used in the preparation of therapeutic fractions ?

ASSAY METHODS

Protein assay has become almost exclusively immunological. All other methods are disappearing as their lack of specificity yields data of decreasing value in clinical situations. Unless one can single out one single protein by one particular chemical technique, as happens in the case of iron in hemoglobin, there is little prospect for any but immunological methods. Nowadays, a total protein assay based on some general chemical or physical property common to all proteins is more difficult to interpret correctly than one which singles out a single protein from a complex milieu by an immunospecific reaction.

The development of immunology through a combination of adsorbent techniques, either in columns, on beads or on the tube-wall, and combined with the introduction of new tricks, such as the laser, for detection of protein-antibody precipitates has pushed the limits of detection to the molecular level. In this workshop some papers will deal with quantitative aspects of laser-nephelometry in antigen-antibody reactions. Isotope (Radio-Immuno Assay, RIA) or enzyme detection (Enzyme - Immuno Assay, EIA; Enzyme Linked Immuno Sorbent Assay, ELISA) methods provide excellent quantitative techniques but require more reagents and equipment. Lastly, separation according to mobility isolates polymorphic forms of the same protein or enzyme and yields interesting clinical information.

It is impossible to find anything more specific and more accurate than an antigen-antibody reaction, the biological material being analysed with a selective biological tool devised by the living organism itself. We see no way of designing a more specific tool. As far as comparisons go, we could compare immunology to atomic absorption which also detects and quantitates a quality inherently characteristic of the individual basic structure of a specific chemical. Who could imagine a better parameter than such an inborn and authentic characteristic ? In brief, then, proteins provide a challenge because of their endless diversity. A century of immunology has demonstrated that the best weapon against such proteins, either in the patient or in the laboratory, is the immunoglobulin, another protein. The correct definition of this reference immunoglobulin is the cornerstone of correct quantitation and identification.

DISCUSSION

The discussion dealt with two problems touched off by this introductory paper, namely the antigenicity of material from animal origin and the use of Freon as a delipidating agent. Hobbs was reluctant to make any major effort for use of animal proteins or other foreign polypeptide material which in the end could turn out to be antigenic, one of the major reasons being the attitude of the American Food And Drug Administration (FDA). To this Peeters replied that insulin is an animal polypeptide and nobody questions its clinical value. Insulin proves that non-human polypeptides can be beneficial. From the delipidation point of view, Hobbs was interested in the therapeutic use of Freon-cleared plasma after experimentation on primates. Freon-clearing would favour reuse of large amounts of human material now being thrown away. Ballieux used Freon-delipidated bovine thymus as a substitute for pure thymic hormone. In the course of preparing immunosuppressive factor from thymus, the thymus lipoproteins provided a stumbling block. After Freon treatment heat stable and sterilizable material became available. Animal experimentation in the primate could prove the validity of this approach. At this point, Hobbs proposed monospecific columns against Clq or reumatoid factor to strip plasma of small immune complexes in cryoprotein disease. This would mean that the patient could receive back his own plasma thus achieving a major saving of human plasma. Intorp picked up the idea of thermostable tissue material and mentioned the problems connected with preparation of heat stable and ethanol-soluble tissue antigens characteristic of vascular tissue.

The Clinical Relevance of Autoimmune Reactions in Renal Disease

Hans W. Intorp

Münster, Germany

Autoimmune reactions are defense mechanisms directed against the body's own organs and tissues. They can be elicited by hetero-,iso- or auto-immunization with immunologically or biochemically defined antigens. These antigens are, with very few exceptions, tissue-specific components present in one tissue but absent from all others. These antigens immunologically characterize the organ or tissue in which they are located.

Immunization can be induced in animals by injection of purified antigenic material incorporated in Freund's adjuvant. During a disease process cell necrosis or destruction can cause continuous liberation of antigens. The trigger mechanism could well be an infection, either bacterial or viral, which may have an adjuvant effect on antigenic activity. The immunization process usually stimulates both humoral and cellular immune reactions which can be demonstrated by immunological techniques such as hemagglutination, complement fixation, precipitation, immunofluorescence, radio-immunoassay, migration-inhibition and lymphocyte stimulation tests. Depending on the structure of the antigen, the intensity of the stimulation and the degree of exposure of the antigen to T- and B-lymphocytes, either humoral antibody production or a cellular immune reaction could prevail. Numerous studies during the past ten years have revealed that in some autoimmune processes humoral immune reactions predominate, while the cellular reactions are more prominent in others. Together with these autoimmune reactions come clinical symptoms which characterize the localization and severity of the disease.

Although autoimmune reactions occur rather frequently only some give rise to autoimmune disease. In the early sixties Witebsky put forward a set of criteria which have now been generally accepted in the definition of autoimmune diseases (42). To classify a pathological process as an autoimmune disease, the stimulating antigen must be immunologically characterized. The tissue specific antigen must be able to elicit humoral or cellular autoimmune reactions which can be demonstrated by standard immunological techniques. The autoimmune reactions must cause pathological changes in animals. Furthermore these autoimmune reactions should be reproducible in other experimental animals by transfer of autoantibodies or immuno-competent cells. Although there is little doubt that in older age groups autoimmune reactions occur more frequently as consequences of other diseases, there are several well known pathological processes which,according to Witebsky's criteria, can be classified as autoimmune diseases. These include autoimmune thyroiditis,allergic encephalomyelitis, autoimmune orchitis, autoimmune glomerulonephritis, autoimmune adrenalitis, myasthenia gravis, autoimmune hemolytic anemia, idiopathic thrombocytopenic purpura, systemic lupus erythematosus, and chronic active hepatitis.

The classical example is autoimmune thyroiditis, better known as Hashimoto's thyroiditis (29,39,44). Allergic encephalomyelitis, which may occur in man, has been induced in experimental animals by Paterson (25). Furthermore, the studies of Voisin (41), Rumke (30) Shulman and others (34) reveal that autoantibodies against semen and testis play an important role in autoimmune orchitis. The intensive studies of Dameshek, Schwartz and their colleagues (32, 33) have proved that autoimmune hemolytic anemias can be induced with auto-antibodies against surface antigens on erythrocytes. In idiopathic thrombocytopenic purpura autoantibodies against thrombocytic antigens also have a cytotoxic effect if complement is present (3,6,21). Not only in autoimmune thyroiditis but also in autoimmune adrenalitis, cellular immune reactions, as evidenced by the activity of T-lymphocytes in these diseases, play a far more important role in pathogenesis than do humoral immune reactions (19,38,43). With the aid of modern immunological techniques it has been shown that in more than 50% of cases of idiopathic adrenalitis autoimmune reactions can be demonstrated (17). By contrast, autoimmune reactions account for only about 8% of the various forms of acute glomerulonephritis. In this disease, however, autoantibody formation causes rapidly progressive lesions in the glomerular basement membrane (40). Other well established autoimmune diseases where autoantibodies play an important role are systemic lupus erythematosus (18) and myasthenia gravis (24). In other illnesses, such as chronic active hepatitis, pemphigus vulgaris and rheumatoid arthritis, autoimmune reactions have been demonstrated but experimental evidence is still needed before they can be classified as autoimmune diseases (1,5,20)

Although detailed information has been obtained in many instances the pathogenesis of autoimmune reactions is still poorly understood. Various mechanisms may be important in this connection. A slight change in antigenic structure of the auto-antigen may result in autoantibody formation. Alternatively the antigens, usually hidden away from the immune system, may become exposed and so induce autoimmune reactions. Another explanation could be that tolerance against the body's own structure breaks down so that mechanisms of self recognition fail. This might explain the higher frequency of autoimmune reactions in older people. In addition, individual differences in immunological reactivity have been considered as etiological factors in autoimmune reactions. Thus "high responders" have been distinguished from "low responders". This theory is based on the observation that in groups of "high responders" autoimmune reactions can frequently be demonstrated and are directed against various tissue specific antigens. Occasionally a combination of 2 or more autoimmune diseases has been described in one such individual(31).

EXPERIMENTAL LESIONS

(i) Glomerulonephritis. In order to study the clinical relevance of autoimmune reactions and diseases, our group has been engaged in immunological investigations dealing with glomerular and tubular renal disease. An experimental model has been developed in which typical clinical symptoms and pathological changes of the mesangio-proliferative form of glomerulonephritis are exhibited (7,8,9). Rabbits were immunized with purified fractions of glomerular basement membrane. This resulted in the formation of circulating autoantibodies which could be demonstrated by complement fixation, double diffusion gel-precipitation and indirect immunofluorescence tests. To determine whether or not autoantibody production, already demonstrated by Stebley (35) and by Dixon and his group (4,15), is accompanied by cellular immune reactions, numerous blood specimens from the immunized animals were examined by the migration inhibition test.

The experiments revealed that a few weeks after autoantibody production had started, cellular immune reactions could be demonstrated. This suggests that in the chronic stage of the disease cellular immune reactions may play an additional role in mesangioproliferative glomerulonephritis. By using autologous renal tissue preparations in migration inhibition tests the autoimmune nature of these reactions was demonstrated. In direct immunofluorescence tests performed with the immunized animal's own renal tissue, linear deposits were found at the glomerular basement membrane. The pattern was comparable to the linear immunofluorescence observed in rapidly progressing glomerulonephritis and Goodpasture's syndrome. When sections of the kidneys from immunized animals were examined microscopically and electron-microscopically, pathological findings characteristic of mesangioproliferative glomerulo-nephritis were observed.

(ii) Renal Tubular Necrosis. In contrast to the numerous studies on glomerular renal disease, investigations dealing with autoimmune reactions of the tubular system are rather scarce. In the early seventies Stebley and Rudofsky (36,37) induced tubular necrosis by injecting experimental animals with kidney preparations containing glomerular as well as tubular material. The observed diffuse round cell infiltrates were taken as evidence for the immunopathogenesis of this disease. Further studies on the immunological reactions of the tubular system revealed that as in glomerular renal disease, heterologous immune complex phenomena and autoimmune reactions with antibodies to tubular basement membrane could be demonstrated. Klassen et al. (11,12) observed granular immunofluorescence in the proximal tubules of rabbits immunized with homologous renal tissue preparations. Using the indirect immunofluorescence technique, antibodies against cytoplasmic antigens of cells from the proximal tubules could be identified. Similar findings were reported by Andres (unpublished) in patients suffering from systemic lupus erythematosus.

To determine whether or not the tubular system can be involved in autoimmune reactions, our group has studied immunological reactions in pyelonephritis and other renal tubular diseases. Rabbits were immunized with heterologous renal tissue preparations free of glomerular structures. They formed antibodies against cytoplasmic antigens of tubular cells which also reacted with homologous structures located in the proximal tubules of the rabbit kidney. These findings were confirmed by double diffusion gel precipitation tests, using different fractions of the tubular system. Immunohistological studies of kidney sections from the immunized animals revealed granular fluorescence of the tubular basement membrane in some rabbits. Other authors have also reported experimental studies in which autoantibodies were formed against antigens of the proximal tubules (13,14). Experimental animals immunized with purified tubular basement membrane preparations produced antibodies which induced linear fluorescence at the tubular basement membrane. These observations indicate that at least one antigen of the tubular system is located in the basement membrane. Occasionally, indirect immunofluorescence tests indicated the formation of antibodies which were directed against a common antigen present at the basement membrane of both tubules and glomeruli.

Further studies were undertaken to determine whether immunization with tubular antigenic fractions causes cellular immune reactions too. Several migration inhibition tests indicated that in tubular autoimmune processes cellular immune reactions can also be demonstrated. At present, differentiation between antigens which stimulate cellular immune reactions is not possible. The results obtained in animal experiments suggest that not only humoral but also cellular autoimmune reactions against tubular antigens may occur. Interestingly, in patients with renal transplants, Klassen's group (10,12) found autoantibodies directed against the tubular basement membrane. These findings indicate that antigens in the tubular basement membrane of donor kidneys stimulate autoantibody formation in the recipent. Although numerous studies of renal glomerular disease have shown that autoimmune

WILLIAM F. MAAG LIBRARY
YOUNGSTOWN STATE UNIVERSITY

reactions are responsible in many instances for glomerular lesions, the relevance of autoimmune reactions in renal tubular disease is not yet clear.

(iii) Pyelonephritis. To study possible roles of autoimmune mechanisms in pyelonephritis, the commonest renal disease in man, our group carried out experiments using the method described by Prat and Hatala (27). When chronic pyelonephritis was induced in rabbits and rats, antibodies directed against the infecting microorganism were produced. The titers depended largely on the concentration of injected bacteria but it made no difference whether virulent or formalin inactivated bacteria were used. In addition, high antibody titers were obtained no matter which route of injection was used (16). Formation of antibodies against infecting bacteria has also been described in human pyelonephritis (22, 23). On the basis of numerous clinical studies of serum antibody titers it is possible to determine the microorganism responsible for a primary infection (22,28). Furthermore, in chronic pyelonephritis new infections can be differentiated from reinfections by the same bacteria. However, changes in titer give no indication of the degree of activity of an infective process (2, 26, 28).

During the last 5 years our group has made an analysis of antibody formation in chronic experimental pyelonephritis. These studies showed that cross reacting antibodies are produced. The antibodies elicited by intravenous injections of bacteria react not only with the infecting micro-organisms but also with a kidney specific antigen of the experimental animal. These antibodies are found rather frequently in the serum of infected rabbits. To determine whether these are true autoantibodies, special experiments were carried out in which the antigens were tested for their reaction with preparations from the uninfected right kidney of the experimental animal itself. In all experiments the autoimmune nature of this reaction was demonstrated. In addition other antibodies were detected which were directed against an antigen common to the kidney and liver. Analytical studies indicated that this common antigen is located in mitochondria. These findings were confirmed in several blind tests.

To clarify the mechanism responsible for autoimmune reactions in experimental pyelonephritis, further studies were undertaken. It turned out that the traumatic alteration induced by temporary ligation of one ureter is important for autoantibody formation. Injections of microorganisms alone cause production of antibodies against the infecting bacteria but not against renal tissue. In order to localise kidney antigens in tissue, fluorescence microscopic studies were performed. These experiments revealed that kidney specific antigens are present in the tubular structures of the renal cortex and medulla. The reaction patterns differ slightly, depending on the specificity of the antisera used for the study. Other immunofluorescence studies indicated that immunization of rabbits with tubular antigens generates autoantibodies which also react with infecting microorganisms. This observation shows that there is formation of cross-reacting antibodies following immunization with tubular antigens which apparently have their counterpart at the surface of the Escherichia coli strain used in these experiments.

Further immunological studies are needed to determine whether a similar pathogenetic mechanism is of relevance in human chronic pyelonephritis. Autoimmune reactions could help to explain why cases of chronic pyelonephritis, in which bacteruria is absent, show a tendency to progress for months or even years. In these instances a self perpetuating mechanism could be responsible for progressively increasing kidney insufficiency.

ACKNOWLEDGEMENT : These studies were supported by the Ministerium für Wissenschaft und Forschung des Landes Nordrhein-Westfalen.

REFERENCES

1. Beutner, E. H. (1969) Autoimmunity in pemphigus and pemphigoid diseases. In "Textbook of Immunopathology" (Miescher, P.A. and Mueller-Eberhard, H.J., Eds.), volume II, Grune and Straten, New York pp.655-664.

2. Brühl, P. and Tunn, W. Immunologische Aspekte der Pyelonephritis - die Bedeutung der unspezifischen Infektresistenz und der Immunität. Der Urologe 1,37 (1967).

3. Dausset, J. and Nenna, A. Présence d'une leucagglutinine dans le sérum d'un cas d'agranulocytose chronique. Sangre (Barc.) 24, 410 (1953).

4. Dixon, F.J., McPhaul, J.J. and Lerner, R.A. The contribution of kidney transplantation to the study of glomerulonephritis. The recurrence of glomerulonephritis in renal transplants. Transpl.Proc. 1, 194 (1969).

5. Doniach, D. Autoimmunity in liver diseases. Progr.Clin.Immunol. 1, 45 (1972).

6. Harrington, W.J., Hollingsworth, J.W. and Moore, C.V. Demonstration of a thrombocytopenic factor in the blood of patients with thrombocytopenic purpura. J.Lab. Clin.Med. 38, 1 (1951).

7. Igelmann, H.J., Intorp, H.W., Gruber, H. and Losse, H. Die Bedeutung zellulärer Immunreaktionen bei den rapidprogressiven Glomerulonephritiden (in press).

8. Intorp, H.W., Igelmann, H.J. and Losse, H. Immunologische Studien zur Pathogenese der Autoimmunglomerulonephritiden. (in press).

9. Intorp, H.W. Mönninghoff, W. and Loew, H. Nierenautoantikörper und ihre Bedeutung bei der Nierentransplantation. Med.Welt. 24,687 (1973).

10. Klassen, J., Andres, G.A., Brennan, J.C. and McCluskey, R.T. An immunologic renal tubular lesion in man. Clin.Immunol. Immunopathol.1,69 (1972).

11. Klassen, J. McCluskey, R.T. and Milgrom, F. Non-glumerular renal disease produced in rabbits by immunization with homologous kidney. Am.J.Path.63,333 (1971)

12. Klassen, J. and Milgrom F. Autoimmune concomitants of renal allografts. Transplant.Proc. 1, 605 (1969).

13. Lehmann, D.H., Marquardt, H., Wilson, C.B. and Dixon, F.J. Specificity of autoantibodies to tubular and glomerular basement membrane induced in guinea pigs. J.Immunol.112, 241 (1974).

14. Lehmann, D.H. Wilson, L.B. and Dixon, F.J. Interstitial nephritis in rats immunized with heterologous tubular basement membrane. Kidney Int.5, 187 (1974)

15. Lerner, R., Glassock, R.J. and Dixon, F.J. The role of antiglomerular basement membrane antibodies in the pathogenesis of human glomerulonephritis. J.Exp.Med. 126, 989 (1967).

16. Loew, H., Ritzerfeld, W., Christ, H. and Losse, H. (1972) Untersuchungen über den E. Coli-Antikörpertiter bei der experimentellen Pyelonephritis. In "Pyelonephritis" (Losse H.H. und Kienitz, M. Eds.), Vol.III, Thieme Verlag, Stuttgart pp.117-122.

17. Mead, R.K. Autoimmune Addison's disease. New Eng.J.Med. 266, 583 (1962).

18. Miescher, P.A. and Paronetto, F. (1969) Systemic lupus erythematosus. In"textbook of Immunopathology" (Miescher, P.A. and Mueller-Eberhard, H.J., Eds.) Vol.II, Grune and Stratton, London. pp 675-712.

19. Milgrom, F. and Witebsky, E. Immunological studies on adrenal glands. I.Immunization with adrenals of foreign species. Immunology, Lond. 5, 67 (1962).

20. Milgrom, F., Witebsky, E., Goldstein, R. and Loza, U. Studies on the rheumatoid and related serum factors. II. Relation of anti-human and anti-rabbit gamma globulin factors in rheumatoid arthritis serums.J.Amer.Med.Ass.181,476 (1962).

21. Müller-Eberhard, H.J., Nilsson, U.R., Dalmasso, A.P., Polley, M.J. and Calcott B.A. A molecular concept of immune cytolysis. Arch.Path. 82, 205 (1966).

22. Neter, E., Steinhart, J., Calcagno, P.L. and Rubin, M.I. (1965) Urinary tract infection in children: I. Studies on antiboy response. In "Progress in Pyelonephritis" (Kass, E.H., Ed.) Davis, Philadelphia, pp.129-135.

23. Neter, E., Westphal, O., Lüderitz, O. and Gorzinsky, E.A. The bacterial hemagglutination test for the demonstration of antibodies to enterobacteriaceae. Ann.N.Y.Acad.Sci. 66, 141 (1965).

24. Osserman, K.E. (1969) Myasthenia gravis. In "Textbook of Immunopathology". Miescher, P.A. and Mueller-Eberhard, H.J.Eds.) Vol.II, Grune and Stratton, London, pp.607-623.

25. Paterson, P.Y. Experimental allergic encephalomyelitis and autoimmune disease. Adv.Immunol. 5, 131 (1966).

26. Percival, A., Brumfitt, W. and Louvois, J.D. Serum antibody levels as an indication to clinically inapparent pyelonephritis. Lancet.II, 1027 (1964).

27. Prat, V. and Hatala, M. Experimental hematogenous E. coli pyelonephritis in the rabbit. Acad.Public Praha. pp 7-82 (1967)

28. Ritzerfeld, W., Prat, V. Konickova, L. and Losse, H. Diagnostik von Harnwegsinfekten: Über die Korrelation von Harnwegsinfektion und Antikörpertiter im Tierversuch. Fortschr.Med. 87, 1293 (1969).

29. Roitt, I.M., Campbell, P.N. and Doniach, D. The nature of the thyroid autoantibodies present in patient with Hashimoto's tyroiditis.(Lymphadenoid Goitre) Biochem.J.69, 248 (1958).

30. Rümke, Ph. Autospermagglutinins: A cause of infertility in men. Ann.N.Y.Acad. Sci. 124, 696 (1965)

31. Schiller, K.F.R., Snyder, M. and Valloron, M.B. Gastric, haematological and immunological abnormalities in Hashimoto's thyroiditis. Gut. 8, 582 (1967).

32. Schwartz, R.S. and Costea, N. Autoimmune hemolytic anemia: Clinical correlations and biological implications. Seminar Hemat.3, 2 (1966).

33. Schwartz, R. and Dameshek, W. The treatment of autoimmune hemolytic anemia with 6-mercaptopurine and thioguanine. Blood 19, 483 (1962).

34. Shulman, S., Yantorne, C., Soanes, W.A., Gonder, M.J. and Witebsky, E.Studies on organ specificity. SVI. Urogenital tissues and autoantibodies. Immunology 10, 99 (1966).

35. Steblay, R.W. (1969) Studies on experimental autoimmune glomerulonephritis: their relevance to human diseases. In "International Convocation of Immunology", Karger, Basel/New York, p 286.

36. Steblay, R.W.and Rudofsky, U. Renal tubular disease and autoantibodies against tubular basement membrane induced in guinea pigs. J.Immunol. 107, 589 (1971).

37. Steblay, R.W. and Rudofsky, U. Transfer of experimental autoimmune renal cortical tubular and interstitial disease in guinea pigs by serum. Science 180, 966 (1973).

38. Terplan, K., Witebsky, E. and Milgrom F. Histopathology of adrenals in animals immunized with tissue antigens. Arch.Path.76, 333 (1963).

39. Terplan, K.L., Witebsky, E., Rose, N.R., Paine, J.R. and Egan, R.W. Experimental thyroiditis in rabbits, guinea pigs and dogs, following immunization with thyroid extracts of their own and of heterologous species. Amer.J.Path. 36, 213 (1960).

40. Unanue, E.R. and Dixon, F.J. (1967) Experimental glomerulonephritis: Immunological events and pathogenetic mechanisms. Adv.Immunol. 6,1 (1967).

41. Voisin, G., Delaunay, A. and Barber, M. Sur des lésions testiculaires provoquées chez le cobaye par iso- et auto-sensibilisation. Ann. Inst.Pasteur 81, 48 (1951).

42. Witebsky, E. (1962) Immunologie und klinische Bedeutung der Autoantikörper. In "Verhandlungen der Deutschen Gesellscharft für innere Medizin, Wiesbaden, Kongress". Vol.68, Bergmann, pp.349-362.

43. Witebsky, E. and Milgrom, F. Immunological studies on adrenal glands. II.Immnization with adrenals of the same species. Immunology, Lond. 5,67 (1962).

44. Witebsky, E. Rose, N.R., Terplan, K., Paine, J.R. and Egan, R.W. Chronic thyroiditis and autoimmunization. J.Amer.Med.Ass. 164, 1439 (1957).

DISCUSSION

Discussion of Professor Intorp's paper was again concerned with therapeutic aspects of auto-immune disease. Intorp concentrated his opening remarks on auto-immune diseases of the kidney which appear to result from two processes. First there are diseases mediated predominantly by auto-antibodies specific to some tissue element (eg. glomerular basement membrane) of the kidney. Secondly, there are diseases primarily due to the cytotoxic actions of cellular elements stimulated by the immune process. In either case, suppression of the immune process would prevent the disease. A method of treatment now being introduced in several centres involves plasmapheresis to remove circulating antibodies and immuno-suppression to prevent their production. Within the past two years, several groups in England and France have used plasmapheresis to treat Goodpasture's syndrome (mesangio proliferative nephritis). Intorp had also used plasmapheresis to treat five patients with Goodpasture's syndrome but he agreed with Ballieux that improvements were only temporary. Hobbs also pointed out that this method would require the use of many blood donors. Set against these disadvantages in this instance, Intorp pointed out that Goodpasture's disease is fortunately rare and cannot yet be treated by any other means. Ballieux suggested that this syndrome might also respond to treatment if lymphocytes from affected patients were re-infused after induction in vitro of suppressive activity. This would only become possible, however, if the responsible renal antigen could be isolated in pure form, an objective which has yet to be realised.

Recent Observations on Plasma Proteins Found During Inflammatory Reactions

Robert Engler

Paris, France

Whenever there is an inflammatory reaction in humans or in experimental animals, two types of response are observed. First, there is a local reaction with venous dilatation, accumulation of leucocytes, deposition of fibrin and liberation of lysosomal enzymes, histamine, serotonin, kinins and prostaglandins. Secondly, there is a systemic reaction which comprises not only fever, pain and leucocytosis, but also a very significant increase in the concentration of plasma glycoproteins, the so-called Inflammatory-Reaction-Glycoproteins (IRG) or, as they will be called here, Acute-Phase-Reactants (APR).

Whatever may be the cause of the inflammatory reaction, be it traumatic, chemical, physical, bacterial, viral or neoplastic, the common feature seems to be rupture of lysosomal sacs and the localised release of enzymes. All glycoproteins related to such inflammatory reactions are synthesised in the liver cells. Although they are found under normal circumstances, hepatic synthesis of these proteins is greatly increased during an inflammatory reaction.

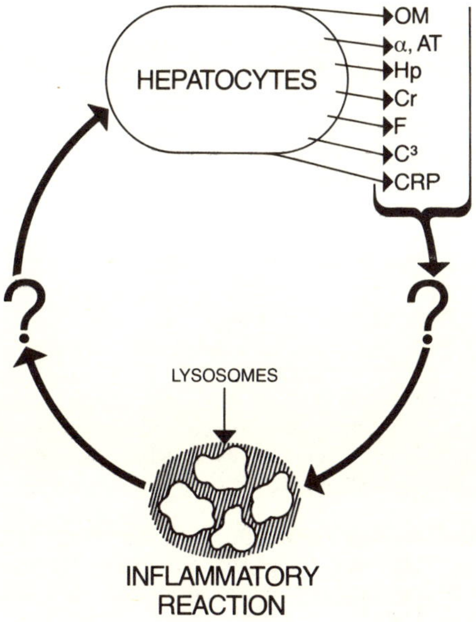

Figure 1. Schematic representation of of substances released by the liver following inflammation of a peripheral tissue. The abbreviations used for AP Reactants are defined in Table I and Figure 2. The stimulants carried in the blood are unknown.

TABLE I

A.P.REACTANT	NORMAL	ACUTE INFLAMMATION
OROSOMUCOIC (OM)	0.6 - 0.9	1.5 - 3.0
α_1 ANTITRYPSIN (α1AT)	2.5 - 4.0	5 - 7
HAPTOGLOBIN (Hp)	0.6 - 1.8	3 - 6
CERULOPLASMIN (Cr)	0.3 - 0.6	1 - 2
FIBRINOGEN (F)	3.0 - 4.0	6 - 10
COMPLEMENT C3 (C3)	1.3 - 1.7	2 - 3
C-REACTIVE PROTEIN (CRP)	0	0.1

Table I : Concentrations (G/l) of certain Acute Phase Reactants (APR) in plasma under normal and acute inflammatory conditions.

In the first figure (Figure 1), are shown schematically a local tissue reaction and the consequent response of the liver cells to inflammation. In Table I are listed the concentrations of glycoproteins found in human plasma normally and during an acute inflammatory reaction. It should be emphasised that C-reactive protein, which can only be found in traces under normal circumstances, can reach concentrations of 0.2 g/l during 24 hours following an acute inflammatory reaction. Although a C-reactive protein exists in the rabbit, none has been reported in rats. The α-2-macroglobulin (α-2-M) can be considered as its equivalent for purposes of diagnosis of the acute inflammatory reaction. In man immunochemical estimates of these plasma proteins permit us to generate profiles characteristic of specific syndromes. If the normal levels of the various proteins are expressed as 100, then, as shown in Figure 2, some proteins show a characteristic change during acute inflammation while a different pattern emerges during sub-acute inflammation.

DIFFICULTIES INVOLVED IN INTERPRETATION OF PLASMA-PROTEIN LEVELS

Two examples can be quoted to illustrate the sort of difficulties involved in interpretation of observations made during episodes of inflammation.

(a) Fibrinogen - During an inflammatory reaction it is quite usual to relate increased rate of red cells sedimentation to plasma fibrinogen concentration. In fact, the fibrinogen molecule is asymmetrical and by a purely mechanical process could favour rouleaux formation and the aggregation of red cells. Obviously, the presence of monoclonal paraprotein leads to the same consequences.

When interpreting rates of red cell sedimentation in the absence of anemia, the doctor should make sure that no corticosteroid therapy is being given. For instance, in children suffering from acute articular rheumatism and showing signs of a very typical acute inflammatory reaction, intensive treatment with corticorsteroids restores to normal in three days both the red cell sedimentation rate and the plasma fibrinogen level. On the other hand, the levels of other APRs, and particularly those of haptoglobin and orosomucoid, remain elevated. It is standard practice to continue such treatment until haptoglobin and orosomucoid levels are again normal. If this is not done, the inflammatory reaction will recur.

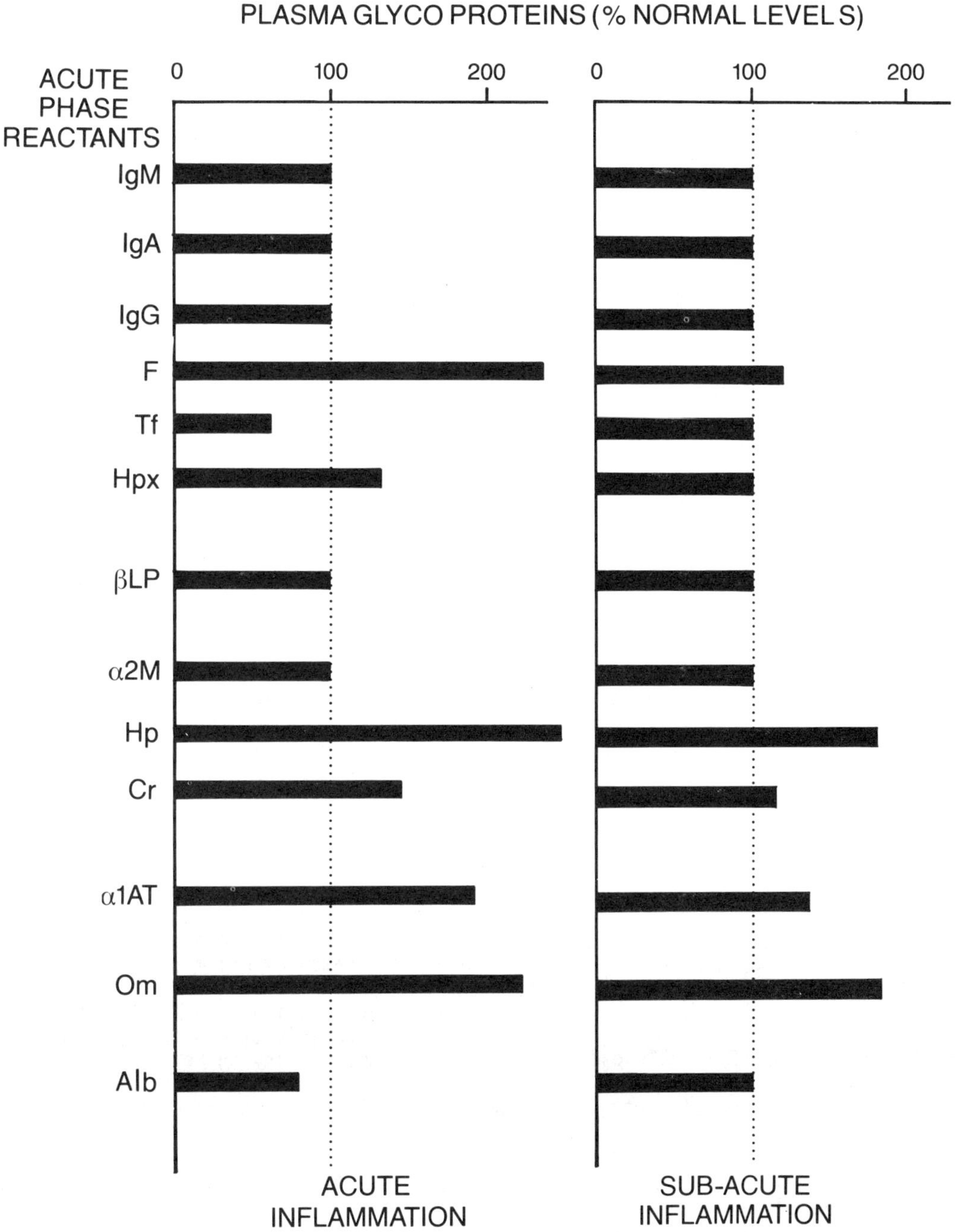

Figure 2. Concentrations, shown as percentages of normal values, of glycoproteins during acute and sub-acute inflammations. Abbreviations refer to those already defined in Table 1 or to immune globulins (IgM, IgA and IgG), Transferrin (Tf), Hemopexin (Hpx), β-lipoproteins (βLP), α2macroglobulins, (α2M) and albumin (Alb).

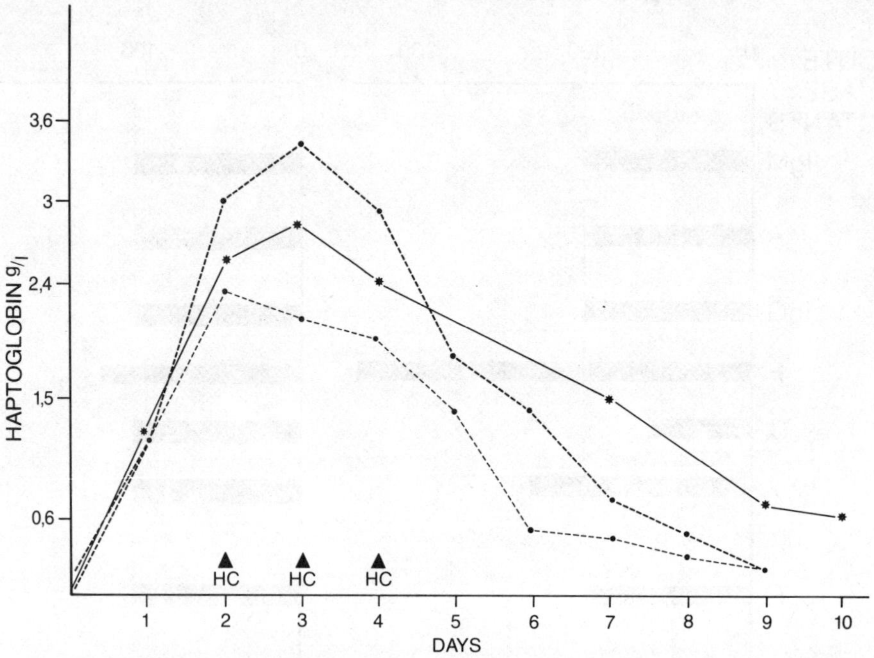

Figure 3. The concentrations (g/l) of haptoglobin in the plasma of individual rabbits are shown after injection at time zero with turpentine. The levels refer to two animals (●.....●) which received no treatment and one (*—— *) injected with hydrocortisone (HC) two, three and four days after receiving turpentine.

Dhermy and I (3) have tried to reproduce this phenomenon in the rabbit. In the first place we isolated fibrinogen and haptoglobin from the rabbit and then, after inducing antibodies to each in the rat, perfected immunochemical methods for their assay. The haptoglobin was purified by the method or Lombart (Personal Communication) in three stages-precipitation with 50-70% saturated ammonium sulphate, and filtration over DEAE-Sephadex-A50 and then over Sephadex-G200. The rabbit fibrinogen was prepared by a technique which involved precipitation with ammonium sulfate at two concentrations (18% and 25% of saturation), precipitation with 2M-phosphate, chromatography on DEAE-cellulose and, finally, chromatography on Sepharose-6B (2).

The concentration of haptoglobin, and of fibrinogen in the plasma of rabbits after induction of an inflammatory reaction with turpentine are shown in Figures 3 and 4. The effects of treatment with corticosteroids are also shown. It is seen that the changes in concentration of these two proteins did not follow the same pattern. Under the influence of repeated injections of hydrocortisone, the fibrinogen level returned to normal while that of haptoglobin followed the same course seen in the untreated animal.

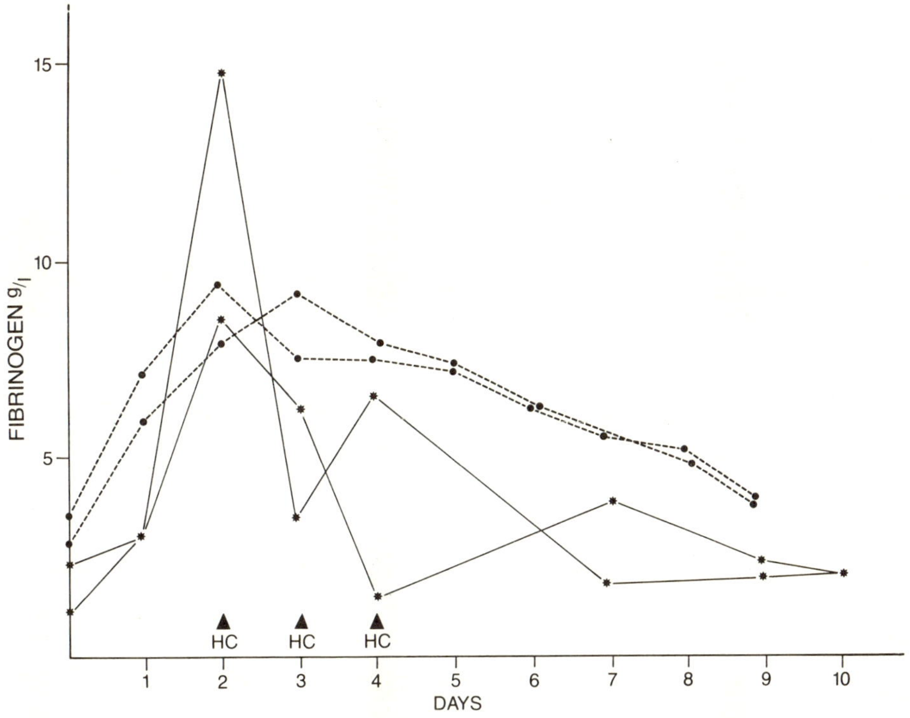

Figure 4. The concentrations (g/l) of fibrinogen in the plasma of two pairs of rabbits are shown after injection at time zero with turpentine. Two rabbits received no other treatment (o.....o) and two (* *) received hydrocortisone (HC) two, three and four days after receiving turpentine.

(b) Haptoglobin. Haptoglobin is a typical APR and during intravascular hemolysis it forms with hemoglobin a complex which is rapidly removed from the circulation, probably by the reticulo-endothelial system. By marking the Hp-Hb complex either with ^{131}I on the haptoglobin fraction or with ^{59}Fe on the hemoglobin fraction, we were able to show that the biological half-life of the complex is one hour and thirty minutes (6). This contrasts with the half-life of free haptoglobin which is three days. The site of catabolism of the Hp-Hb complex is the subject of much controversy. Some consider that it becomes localised in hepatocytes and others think it is removed by reticulo-endothelial cells (5). At any rate, during an episode of intravascular hemolysis little or no haptoglobin is found in the plasma, as shown by immuno-electrophoresis using an anti-haptoglobin serum and by electophoresis on poly-acrylamide gel. In the very frequent cases where intra-vascular hemolysis is associated with an acute inflammatory reaction, a single determination of haptoglobin would not be sufficient. In order to make the complete diagnosis of moderate intravascular hemolysis and acute inflammation, it would also be necessary to determine the orosomucoid level (7).

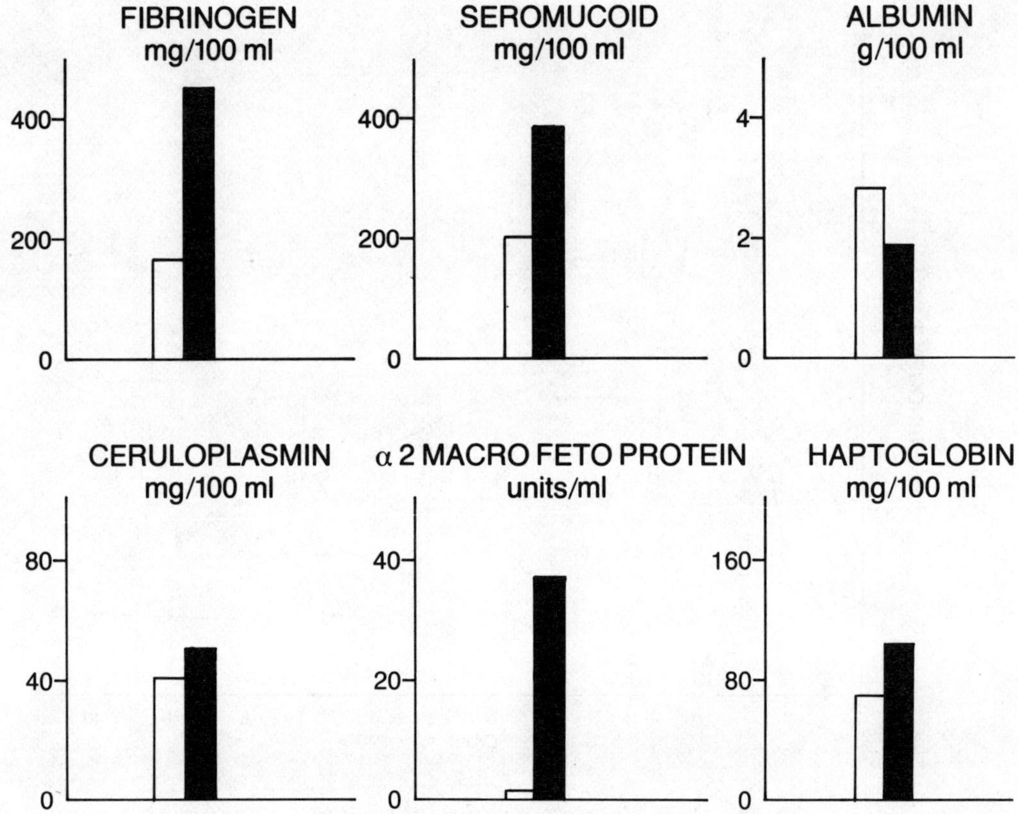

Figure 5. The plasma concentrations of proteins before (open columns) and 24 hrs. after (closed columns) intraperitoneal injection of Leucocyte Endogenous Mediator (LEM). This data was previously presented by Wannamacher et al. (11).

ORIGIN OF THE ENDOGENOUS FACTOR ELEVATING GLYCOPROTEIN LEVELS IN THE INFLAMMATORY REACTION

As early as 1945, Homburger observed that pus derived from a sterile abscess induced by injection of turpentine contains a thermo-labile substance which on intravenous injection increases fibrinogen concentration. In 1964, Borel and his colleagues (1) provided evidence for a factor intermediate between the peripheral tissue in which a granuloma is induced and the liver.

From a healthy rabbit, after sacrifice, the present authors have removed various organs more or less rich in connective tissue (lung, muscle, sub-cutaneous tissue, etc.). Three grams of tissue from each organ were ground in the presence of normal serum at 4°C and then on the following day the soluble components were extracted. Intravenous injection of the soluble extract into a healthy rabbit caused marked increase in concentration of haptoglobin in the plasma. If these results are compared with those following subcutaneous injection of turpentine it is found that the peak of the curve is rapidly reached, within thirty hours, and much more rapidly than after turpentine injection. On the other hand, this increase is more transient for within 48 to 72 hours after injection of the extract, the plasma haptoglobin level is again normal as opposed to the 6 to 8 days taken for the level to fall to normal after induction of an inflammatory reaction, infectious or chemical.

In 1970, Sarcione (9) observed increased incorporation of radioactive amino acids into APRs while perfusing isolated livers with blood drawn from animals during an inflammatory reaction. Of the early mediators of inflammation (histamine, serotonin, and SRS-A, the slow reacting substance of anaphylaxis, etc.), only the prostaglandins were capable on injection into animals of significantly increasing hepatic production of APRs. The PGE_1 - prostaglandins could stimulate haptoglobin biosynthesis in the rabbit's liver through a mechanism involving a decrease in the level of cyclic-AMP. This is interesting but the pharmacological dose of PGE_1-prostaglandins which has to be injected, 30μg/kg, is certainly much greater than the amount of prostaglandin released from an induced experimental granuloma.

Another line of research concerned with leucocytes has emerged in recent years. It can be said, as Gerard Weissmann did, that phagocytosis cannot exist without inflammation. The opposite is also true and it can be concluded that phagocytosis plays a pivotal role in the inflammatory response. In 1968, Darcy observed that after injection of leucocytes or sub-cellular fractions made from them, there was a moderate increase in the α1AP-globulins of rats. In 1971, Eddington (4) showed an increase in biosynthesis of APRs after intraperitoneal injection into rabbits of pyrogenic extracts of leucocytes. After 1972, it became possible to isolate a protein factor called LEM (Leucocyte Endogenous Mediator); it appeared in the supernatent solution after centrifugation of a medium in which phagocytosing polymorphonuclear leucocytes of an animal had been incubated at 37°C for 2 hours. When injected into rats or rabbits, this factor caused an increase in the plasma level of APRs. The effects were the same as those obtained after sub-cutaneous injection of turpentine. With the aid of the isolated perfused liver and the intact animal it was found (11) that LEM promotes transport of amino acids to the liver; stimulates incorporation of radio-labelled orotic acid into hepatic RNA of test animals; and further stimulates biosynthesis of the principal inflammatory reaction glycoproteins (haptoglobin, α2-macroglobulin, ceruloplasmin and fibrinogen) as illustrated in Figure 5. Increased RNA biosynthesis is localised in the ribosomes and precedes by six to eight hours the increased biosynthesis of glycoproteins. LEM seems to act directly on the hepatic cell and its actions do not depend upon cyclic-AMP. The effect of corticosteroid hormones appears to be of a permissive nature. These results have a bearing on the participation of leucocytes in the inflammatory process but neither Seligshom nor ourselves have yet been able to confirm them. Injection into the rabbit of an untreated extract obtained after incubation of 10^8 leucocytes from a peritoneal exudate did not result in any significant increase in levels of plasma haptoglobin or fibrinogen.

BIOLOGICAL FUNCTIONS OF INFLAMMATORY REACTION GLYCOPROTEINS

Like Koj (8), one can conclude that every glycoprotein has its own particular part to play in the very early phases of development of an inflammatory granuloma:

(a) Fibrinogen limits hemorrhage by allowing intra- and extra- vascular coagulation, allows the formation of a matrix on which the fibroblasts can build, and forms a substrate upon which proteolytic enzymes such as plasmin and leucocyte proteins can act. Having anti-coagulant properties, the degradation products of fibrinogen exert a sort of local auto-regulatory metabolic action.

(b) The principal function of haptoglobin is to combine with hemoglobin to form the haptoglobin-hemoglobin complex. This complex possesses peroxidase activity which could play a local role in the generation of collagen and of hydroxyl compounds which inactivate molecules responsible for tissue injury. On the other hand, hemoglobin in the form of the haptoglobin-hemoglobin complex, is more rapidly catabolised by Heme-alpha-methenyl oxygenase.

(c) Ceruloplasmin has oxidase activity and obviously plays a role in the local biosynthesis of serotonin and adrenalin and in the delivery of copper to cytochrome oxidase.

(d) C-reactive protein takes part in the formation of heme-proteins, and particularly of catalase, and activates complement.

(e) α1-anti-trypsin, due to its protease activity, neutralises the neutral proteases released locally at the level of the granuloma.

The common feature of all APRs could be manifested at the level of inactivation of lysosomal enzymes and most particularly of lysosomal cathepsins of the leucocytes. Leucocytosis can be shown to occur only a few hours after a granuloma has been induced in an animal. Increased permeability of the lysosomal membranes of leucocytes and the local release of cathepsin could be, according to Houck, an important stage in the local inflammatory reaction. The haptoglobin, or a glucose moiety attached to this protein, would, according to Snellman (10), inhibit lysosomal B1-cathepsin. The ox's orosomucoid, according to Koj and Allison, inhibits Cathepsin-C and haptoglobin inhibits hemoglobulin proteolysis by cathepsin-D. From rat liver lysosomes we have isolated a fraction which is rich in cathepsin-B1 and have measured its enzymatic activity using BANA (Benzoyl Arginyl Naphthylamide) as substrate. Added in a concentration of 1 mg/ml, purified rat haptoglobin inhibits the activity of this enzyme; rat albumin added under the same condition has no effect. In conclusion, APRs released at the level of the lesion, could be playing the role of inactivators of enzymes liberated by the lysosomes and causing tissue degradation.

REFERENCES

1. Borel, J.P., Mouray, H., Moretti, J.M. and Jayle, M.F. Relation entre le tissu conjonctif et l'haptoglobine sérique. C.R. Acad.Sci.Paris, 259, 3875 (1964).

2. Dhermy, D., Judon, C., Engler, R. and Jayle, M.F. Preparation et dosage immunonéphélométrique du fibrinogène de lapin. Biochimie 58,1311 (1976).

3. Dhermy, D., Judon, C., Engler, R. and Jayle, M.F. Fibrinogen and inflammatory state inflence of hydrocortisone. Thrombosis Research 12, 357 (1978).

4. Eddington, C.L., Uchurch, H.P. and Kamschmidt, R.F. Effect of extracts from rabbit leukocytes on levels of acute phase globulins in rat serum. Proc.Soc.Exp. Biol. 136, 159 (1971).

5. Engler, R., Bescol-Liversac, J. and Moretti, J. Catabolisme du complexe haptoglobine dans le système reticulo-endothelial, C.R. Acad. Sci.Paris, 263D,1636 (1966).

6. Engler, R., Moretti, J. and Jayle, M.F. Catabolisme du complexe haptoglobine-hémoglobine. Bull.Soc. Chim. Biol. 49, 263 (1967).

7. ENGLER, R.,WAKIM,A.,POINTIS J.,RONDEAU, Y., JUDON, C. and JAYLE, M.F. Hémolyse intra-vasculaire. Appreciation par le dosage de l'haptoglobine de l'hémopexine et de l'orosomucoïde. La Nouvelle Presse Médicale 4, 1493 (1975)

8. KOJ, A. (1974) Acute phase reactants their synthesis, turnover and biological significance. In "Structure and function of plasma proteins".(Allison, Ac. Ed.) Vol.1, Plenum Press, London, pg 73.

9. SARCIONE, E.J. (1970) Regulation of plasma α2 (acute phase) globulin synthesis in rat liver. In "Plasma protein metabolism" (Rothschild, Ed.) Academic Press, London, pg 369.

10. SNELLMAN, O and SYLVEN, B. A carbohydrate inhibitor of cathepsin-B activity associated with Haptoglobin. Experientia (Basel) 30, 1114 (1974).

11. WANNEMACHER, R.W., PEKARED, R.S., THOMPSON, W.L., CURNOW, R.T., BEALL, F.A., ZENSER, T.Y., de RUBERTIS, F.R. and BEISEL, W.R. A protein from polymorphonuclear leukocytes (LEM) which affects the rate of hepatic amino-acid transport and synthesis of acute phase globulins. Endocrinology, 96, 651 (1975).

DISCUSSION

From an exchange of views between Dolkart and Engler it appeared important to stress the fact that a protein level reflects both synthesis and degradation. Low levels can be due to excessive destruction as well as to insufficiency of production. The inflammatory reaction may increase synthesis and so absolute values could be confusing. From the clinical point of view, there is need for a parameter that would enable one to follow the rate of an inflammatory reaction without consideration of production and consumption of proteins.

Intorp was able to localize C-reactive proteins (CRP) in atherosclerotic lesions and this induced him to believe that this protein provides evidence for degenerative disease rather than for reaction to an inflammatory process. It was the opinion of Engler, however, that not only CRP but also Hp and orosomucoïd occur as local deposits in some lesions. This does not mean that these proteins form a kind of debris but rather confirms their role as inflammatory reaction proteins. According to Hobbs the cholesterol crystals in such lesions would elicit a reaction of leucocytes which could then synthesize CRP locally in the lesion. Thus the CRP in the plasma would represent overflow from the tissue into the circulation and should be considered the result of such local inflammation. Engler also stressed the possibility of testing serum for degradation products of these inflammatory proteins and believes that such tests could provide an interesting field of application for the new nephelometric techniques.

The Clinical Significance of Sensitive Assays For Human Immunoglobulin - A

H. J. Schuurman, R. E. Ballieux and P. J. J. Van Munster

Utrecht, Holland

Quantitation of immunoglobulins in human body fluids is now an important and widely used diagnostic tool in clinical immunology. Single radial immunodiffusion (16) or techniques of similar sensitivity enable precise quantitative analysis of immunoglobulin levels of each class or even subclass. The detection limit of these assay methods is of the order of 0.02 mg/ml. For the determination of lower concentrations of immunoglobulins radioimmunoassay (RIA) has been introduced. This method has been of value in the quantitation of IgE (2) and of IgA in sera of newborns (28) when conventional methods, due to their low sensitivities, are not suitable. Although a wealth of information is available on methodological aspects of immunoglobulin determination, relatively little attention has been paid to the clinical significance of the detection limits of the various assay methods. This is the more remarkable since, for instance, definition of immunoglobulin-A (IgA) deficiency has been incorrectly based solely on the sensitivity of the radial immunodiffusion technique (1).

Deficiency of serum IgA is the most commonly known immunodeficiency whose incidence in normal population is about 0.1% (8,12,37). Quantitative analysis of IgA in sera of IgA deficient individuals is of utmost importance for, in the absence of IgA, blood or plasma transfusion may give rise to formation of class-specific anti-IgA antibodies. These antibodies, once formed, may cause severe anaphylactoid reactions upon administration of plasma or IgA-containing immunoglobulin preparations (14,21,22,36,39). When IgA is present in low but detectable amounts (by RIA), the formation of class-specific anti-IgA antibodies seems very unlikely (19). In principle, total absence of IgA (absolute IgA deficiency) should be defined as a serum concentration of zero with the restriction that this zero value reflects the total absence of any IgA in the body. It is obvious that this is an unpractical definition. Besides, ability to measure concentrations near absolute zero is questionable in view of practical clinical decisions. A discussion on deficiency of IgA can focus on three different elements, one concerned with the assay (the minimal detection limit), one based on a theoretical biological approach (biological concentration limit) and one concerning clinical aspects (level of clinical significance). In the following paragraphs these three elements will be considered in more detail.

The Minimal Detection Limit

Up to now, RIA or related techniques such as enzyme immunoassay (7) have provided the methods of choice for quantitation of very low concentrations of immunoglobulins. The detection limit of RIA can be optimized either by use of physical models (6,38) or by an experimental approach (27). Under optimal conditions sensitivity mainly depends on the avidity of the antiserum. When an antiserum is used with an avidity of about 8×10^9 L/M the minimal detection limit of an one-step inhibition RIA is about 4 ng IgA (26).

The Biological Concentration Limit

The minimum concentration of IgA in serum which is theoretically possible (biological concentration limit) can be defined as the contribution of a single IgA-secreting cell to the serum IgA concentration. This concentration can be estimated in two ways:

a. From the relation between the number of IgA-containing cells in the bone marrow and the total body pool of monomeric IgA. In man, IgA is heterogeneous in molecular size. Serum IgA is mainly, if not totally, monomeric (23) while dimeric IgA is mainly present in the external secretions. This heterogeneity is reflected by the sites of synthesis: dimeric IgA is synthesized locally in glands and mucosa adjacent to the secretory fluid, whereas monomeric serum IgA is synthesized in the bone marrow (10, 29,32) and to a lesser extent in the spleen and peripheral lymph nodes (3,31).

In a study on 74 children and adults, Vossen (35) observed a log-log linear relation between the total number of IgA-containing cells in the bone marrow and the total body pool of IgA. From this data, it follows that 10^5 IgA-containing cells correspond to a total body pool of 0.20 mg IgA. On the assumption that the plasma volume is 3 L and that 45% of the total IgA body pool is present intravasculary (20,35), it can then be deduced that one IgA-containing plasma cell in the bone marrow corresponds with 0.04 pg IgA/ml in the serum.

b. From the kinetics of immunoglobulin synthesis. Salmon (24) proposed the following formula for the total number of immunologlobulin synthesizing cells (n):

$$n = \frac{\text{immunoglobulin synthesizing rate for the total plasma pool}}{\text{immunoglobulin synthesizing rate for one cell}}$$

The immunoglobulin synthesizing rate for the total plasma pool can be estimated from equations given by Salmon (24) and Nadorp (21):

$$\begin{array}{l}\text{Immunoglobulin synthesizing rate} \\ \text{for the total plasma pool}\end{array} = \text{FCR} \times \text{PV} \times \text{C}$$

FCR = fractional catabolic rate, i.e. the fraction of the intravascular amount of IgA which is catabolized per unit of time. Nadorp (21) has reported a value of 18% of the intravascular pool per day. The FCR is about equal for both subclasses of IgA (18) and does not depend on age (30) or serum IgA concentration (21).

PV = Plasma volume. For adults this volume is approximately 3 L.

C = Serum concentration of IgA.

The immunoglobulin synthesizing rate for one cell can be estimated by analysis of the supernatant fluid during *in vitro* culture of immunoglobulin synthesizing cells. Salmon (24) has estimated this rate to be between 4 and 32 pg/cell/day for tumor cells synthesizing myeloma immunoglobulin. After stimulation of tonsillar lymphocytes with pokeweed mitogen, Janossy et al. (11) have observed a rise in the synthesis of IgM and IgG between the fifth and seventh day of culture. This rise was from 5 to 40 pg/cell/day for IgM and from 10 to 70 pg/cell/day for IgG. Data on polyclonal IgA documented in a equally well-defined way are not available for the time being. Assuming daily production of 30 pg IgA, it follows from the equations given above, that a single IgA synthesizing cell contributes 0.06 pg/ml to the serum concentration of IgA.

These estimates of the biological concentration limit are very similar and both models involve basic assumptions. In the first IgA-containing cells in the bone marrow are considered as the only source of serum IgA. In the second one, data obtained from in vitro experiments are applied to the in vivo situation. In both models the dimeric IgA-synthesizing system is not included. Nevertheless, it can be concluded that the biological concentration limit is very low and far below the minimum level of detection by radio-immunoassay. It is worth mentioning however that it has been claimed (5,13,25) that IgA deficient individuals possess normal numbers of lymphocytes in the blood with membrane-bound IgA. Therefore, the serum IgA in these individuals may come from another source, possibly due to turnover (shedding) of IgA from the membrane of these cells. There are no data on shedding in vivo (15). Data on shedding in vitro, obtained by analysis of the supernatant after culture of radioiodinated lymphocytes (4,17,33,34) vary widely. For the mouse, Melchers et al. (17) have observed values for t 1/2 of membrane-bound IgM of 1-3 h and 10-30 h, according to the cell type. Translation of these data to the in vivo situation may not be valid. So, estimation of the contribution of shed immunoglobulin to the serum IgA concentration has to be limited to calculation of the upper limit of the amount of membrane-bound IgA shed per volume of plasma. Assuming a total number of 10^7 IgA-bearing lymphocytes in blood (35), an amount of 10^5 immunoglobulin molecules on the surface of a single cell (9), and a plasma volume of 3 L, this estimate is about 0.1 ng/ml. From this value it can be speculated that the biological concentration limit, at least for IgA deficient individuals with normal numbers of peripheral blood lymphocytes with membrane bound IgA but with a defect in secretion of IgA from IgA-synthesizing cells, is much higher (ca.10-100 pg/ml) than the concentration limit calculated on the basis of secretion by a single IgA-synthesizing cell.

The Level of Clinical Significance

The major importance of an assay for IgA in serum of IgA deficient individuals is its predictive value in the formation of class-specific antibodies. So the level of clinical significance can be defined as the serum IgA concentration below which IgA cannot be recognized any more as "self". This definition is proposed with the restriction that all IgA present in the body is represented in the serum.

Data from the literature may illustrate further the level of clinical significance and indicate its value. Van Munster et al. (19) studied 27 IgA deficient adults (diagnosed by a serum IgA level below 0.02 mg IgA/ml). Either circulating IgA (15/27) using RIA with a detection limit of about 50 ng IgA/ml, or class-specific anti-IgA antibodies (12/27) proved to be detectable in the serum of these individuals. In contrast to this observation, Vyas et al. (37) reported a large proportion (45%) of adult sera without any detectable IgA or antibodies. In the latter study a haemagglutination test with a detection limit of about 500 ng IgA/ml was used for the assay of IgA. Remarkably, in the serum of 17 IgA deficient children aged between 4 and 12 years, IgA could be detected (using the RIA mentioned) in the absence of any detectable anti-IgA antibody; for one child of this group, serum anti-IgA in the presence of circulating IgA became detectable by titration RIA at the age of 11 years (Van Munster, unpublished observations).

From this important preliminary observation and the findings mentioned above it can be speculated that the level of clinical significance lies above the detection limit of the IgA RIA (about 50 ng IgA/ml) and below that of the haemagglutination (500 ng IgA/ml); a further optimization of the sensitivity of the IgA-RIA is not indicated.

CONCLUSIONS

Knowledge is too limited at this moment to allow for a firmly based definition of IgA deficiency. It is our hope that this annotation may stimulate further discussion and may contribute to future investigations on IgA deficient individuals. In particular, studies on IgA deficient children will be of importance, since the results may eludicate some aspects of the formation of class-specific anti-IgA anti-bodies.

ACKNOWLEDGEMENT

We wish to express our gratitude to Dr. F.H.J. Gmelig Meyling for helpful and stimulating discussions on this subject.

REFERENCES

1. Ammann, A.J. and Hong, R. Selective IgA deficiency: presentation of 30 cases and a review of the literature. Medicine (Baltimore) 50, 223 (1971).

2. Bennich, H. and Johansson, S.G.O. Structure and functions of human Immunoglobulin E. Adv. Immunol. 13, 1 (1971)

3. Bernier, G.M. and Cebra, J.J. Frequency distribution of α, γ, κ and λ polypeptide chains in human lymphoid tissues. J. Immunol. 95, 246 (1965)

4. Cone, R.E., Marchalonis, J.J. and Rolley, R.T. Lymphocyte membrane dynamics. Metabolic release of cell surface proteins. J.Exp.Med. 134, 1373 (1971).

5. Delespesse, G., Gausset, Ph., Cauchie, Ch. and Govaerts, A. Cellular aspects of selective IgA deficiency. Clin. Exp. Immunol. 24, 273 (1976).

6. Ekins, R.P., Newman, G.B. and O'Riordan, J.L.H. (1968) Theoretical aspects of "saturation" and radioimmunoassay. In "Radioisotopes in medicine: in vitro studies" (Hayes, R.L. Goswitz, F.A. & Pearson Murphy, B.E., Eds.), U.S. Atomic Energy Comm., Oak Ridge, pp 59-100.

7. Engvall, E. and Perlmann, P. Enzyme-linked immunosorbent assay (ELISA). Quantitative assay of immunoglobulin G. Immunochemistry 8, 871 (1971).

8. Frommel, D., Moullec, J., Lambin, P. and Fine, J.M. Selective serum IgA deficiency. Frequency among 15,200 French blood donors. Vox Sang. 25, 513 (1973).

9. Greaves, M.F., Owen, J.J.T. and Raff, M.C. (1973) T. and B lymphocytes: origins, properties and roles in immune responses, Excerpta Medica, Amsterdam.

10. Hijmans, W., Schuit, H.R.E. and Hulsink-Hesselink, E. An immunofluorescence study on intracellular immunoglobulins in human bone marrow cells. Ann.N.Y. Acad.Sci. 177, 290 (1971).

11. Janossy, G., Gomez de la Concha, E., Luquetti, A., Snajdr, M.J. Maxdal, M.J.and Platts-Mills, T.A.E. T. cell regulation of immunoglobulin synthesis and proliferation in pokeweed (Pa-1) stimulated human lymphocyte cultures. Scand.J.Immunol. 6, 109 (1977).

12. Koistinen, J. Selective IgA deficiency in blood donors. Vox Sang.29, 192 (1975)

13. Lawton, A.R., Royal S.A., Self, K.S. and Cooper, M.D. IgA determinants on B lymphocytes in patients with deficiency of circulating IgA.J.Lab.Clin.Med. 80, 26 (1972).

14. Leikola, J., Koistinen, J., Lehtinen, M. and Virolainen, M. IgA induced anaphylactic transfusion reactions: a report of four cases. Blood 42, 111 (1973).

15. Loor, F. (1977). Structure and dynamics of the lymphocyte surface. In "B and T cells in immune recognition" (Loor, F.O Roelants, G.E., Eds.) Wiley,London pp153-189.

16. Mancini, G., Carbonara, A.O. and Heremans, J.F. Immunochemical quantitation of antigens by sinble radial immunodiffusion. Immunochemistry 2, 235 (1966).

17. Melchers, F., Cone, R.E., von Boehmer, H. and Sprent, J. Immunoglobulin turnover in B lymphocyte subpopulations. Eur.J.Immunol.5, 382 (1975).

18. Morell, A., Skvaril, F. Noseda, G. and Barandun, S. Metabolic properties of human IgA subclasses. Clin.Exp.Immunol.13,521 (1975)

19. Van Munster, P.J.J., Nadorp, J.M.S.M. and Schuurman, H.J. Human antibodies to immunoglobulin A (IgA). A radioimmunological method for differentiation between anti-IgA antibodies and IgA in the serum of IgA deficient individuals. J. Immunol.(Methods) 22, 233 (1978).

20. Nadorp, J.H.S.M., Voss, M. Buys, W.C., Van Munster, P.J.J., van Tongeren, J. H.M. Aalberse, R.F. and Van Loghem, E. The significance of the presence of anti-IgA antibodies in individuals with an IgA deficiency.Eur.J.Clin.Invest. 3, 317 (1973).

21. Nadorp, J.H.S.M. Immuunglobuline A en immuunglobulin A deficientie. Metaboklinische en immunogenetische aspecten. Thesis, Nijmegen, (1974).

22. Pineda, A.A. and Taswell, H.F. Transfusion reactions associated with anti-IgA antibodies: report of four cases and review of the literature. Transfusion , 15, 15 (1975).

23. Radl, J., Swart, A.C.W.and Mestecky, J. The nature of polymeric serum IgA in man. Proc.Soc.Exp.Biol.Med. 150, 482 (1975).

24. Salmon, S.E. Immunoglobulin synthesis and tumor kinetics of multiple myeloma. Semin.Hematol. 10, 135 (1973).

25. Schiff, R.I. Buckley, R.H., Gilbertsen, R.B. and Metzgar, R.S. Membrane receptors and in vitro responsiveness of lymphocytes in human immunodeficiency.J. Immunol.112, 376 (1974)

26. Schuurman, H.J. and de Ligny, C.L. Experimental optimization of the detection limit of one-step solid phase radioimmunoassay. Clin.Chim.Acta 89, 191 (1978)

27. Schuurman, H.J. Solid phase radioimmunoassay of immunoglobulin A.Studies on the detection limit of three assay systems. Thesis, Utrecht (1977).

28. Schuurman, H.J., Hagenaars, A.M. and Zegers, B.J.M. Cord serum levels of IgM, IgA, and α-fetoprotein and their interrelationships. Clin.Chim.Acta.79, 363 (1977).

29. Skvaril, F. and Morell, A. Distribution of IgA subclasses in sera and bone marrow plasma cells of 21 normal individuals. Adv.Exp.Med.Biol. 45, 433 (1974)

30. Stiehm, E.R., Vaerman, J.P. and Fudenberg, H.H. Plasma infusions in immunologic deficiency states: metabolic and therapeutic studies. Blood 28, 918 (1966).

31. Tomasi, T.B.,Jr. Secretory immunoglobulins. New Engl.J.Med. 287,500 (1972).

32. Turesson, I. Distribution of immunoglobulin containing cells in human bone marrow and lymphoid tissues. Acta Med.Scand. 199,293 (1976).

33. Vitetta, E.S. and Uhr, J.W. Immunoglobulins and alloantigens on the surface of lymphoid cells. Biochem.Biophys.Acta. 415, 253 (1975).

34. Vitetta, E.S. and Uhr, J.W. Cell surface immunoglobulin. V. Release from murine splenic lymphocytes. J.Exp.Med. 136, 676 (1972).

35. Vossen, J.M.J.J. The development of the B immune system in man. Thesis, Leiden, (1975).

36. Vyas, G.N., Perkins, H.A. and Fudenberg, H.H. Anaphylactoid transfusion reactions associated with anti-IgA. Lancet ii, 312 (1968).

37. Vyas, G.N., Perkins, H.A., Wang, Y.M. and Basantani, G.K. Healthy blood donors with selective absence of immunoglobulin A: prevention of anaphylactic transfusion reactions caused by antibodies to IgA. J.Lab.Clin.Med. 85,838 (1975).

38. Yalow, R.S. and Berson,S.A. (1968) General principles of radioimmunoassay. In "Radioisotopes in medicine : in vitro studies" (Hayes, R.L. Goswitz, F.A. and Pearson Murphy, B.E., Eds.) U.S. Atomic Energy Comm. Oak Ridge, pp 7-39.

39. Wells, J.V.,Buckley, R.H.,Schanfield, M.S. and Fudenberg, H.H. Anaphylactic reactions to plasma infusions in patients with hypogammaglobulinemia and anti-IgA antibodies. Clin. Immunol. Immunopathol. 8, 265 (1977).

DISCUSSION

Dolkart brought up the problem of denaturation of protein during extracorporeal circulation. According to data mentioned by Hobbs 100 nanogram/ml of pure anti A IgM would be sufficient to hemolyse 50% of the red cells. Ballieux did not see how one can relate amounts of protein to function. Neither is it exactly known how low the level of IgE has to go in order to avoid symptoms. Nor is it known, for instance, what level of IgA is required in order to protect from polio. It is probable that the IgA bearing lymphocytes of IgA deficient individuals shed their membrane-bound IgA into the plasma and this mechanism is responsible for the very low IgA level found in immuno-deficient patients. An anaphylactic reaction occurs in these patients when they receive a gamma globulin preparation. It is suspected that the patients have circulating antigens which form antigen/antibody complexes with the injected immunoglobulins, and that this causes the anaphylactic reactions. This situation is analogous to the side effects of gamma globulin injected into SLE patients and which are likewise due to antibody activity in the injected gamma globulin.

Peeters mentioned that cells in culture do not produce their proteins in a continuous process but in an cyclic process which follows a circadian rhythm of about 24 hours. The proteins arise in waves. Could this have a bearing on the situation described ? Ballieux believes that the half life of an immunoglobulin is much longer than the biological cycle of the cell. However, Dolkart and Hobbs mentioned the existence of hormonal waves that could regulate an entire cell population and cause such rhythmical effects on plasma levels, especially in the case of short-lived proteins.

Some Industrial Aspects of Plasma Protein Production

Rene de Vreker

Costa Mesa, U.S.A.

During 1977 about six million litres of plasma will be fractionated throughout the world. Most current industrial fractionation procedures are based on that described by Cohn using ethanol as a protein-precipitating agent. Ether fractionation is possible but involves a considerable fire hazard and is no longer used. Ammonium sulfate is used by at least one major manufacturer but necessitates the disposal of large amounts of the precipitant. Rivanol has been used in association with ammonium sulfate but its removal from the final product cannot be guaranteed. Hydroxy-ethyl-starch has been used during preparation of immune globulins for intravenous injection but, again, it is difficult to remove from the final product and can cause allergic reactions. Polymers such as polyethylene glycol (PEG) and polypropylene glycol (PPG) have been used for fractionation of plasma in the laboratory but no one has yet used them industrially. Gel filtration has been used but poses the risk of infection which cannot be prevented, as it can in the laboratory, by addition of antiseptic agents.

Alcohol precipitation under various conditions of temperature, pH and ionic strength has proved most effective for plasma fractionation on an industrial scale. Techniques are now available, or are being developed, to improve the method. These techniques allow abbreviation of the existing process to obtain specific proteins more efficiently; denaturation of other proteins while allowing maximum separation of albumin; the handling of very large volumes of reactants at low temperature; reduction from hours to minutes of the period needed for sedimentation of precipitates; and other improvements. Against this background of very brief details it is possible to consider what has been achieved by plasma fractionation and what might be achieved in the future.

As illustrated in the adjoining Figure, the first product obtained from frozen plasma is CRYOPRECIPITATE, an easily prepared derivative still used in the treatment of Hemophilia "A". Further concentration of this fraction yields Factor VIII preparations still capable of correcting deficiencies in patients with Hemophilia "A" but no longer able to correct defects in patients with Von Willebrand's disease. From the remaining supernatent solution, the PROTHROMBIN COMPLEX, including Factor IX, is separated by adsorption onto gels such as DEAE Sephadex or Tricalcium phosphate; Factor IX is used in the treatment of Hemophilia "B". In the first fraction (I) then obtained by alcohol precipitation is FIBRINOGEN which is no longer used therapeutically. The next fraction (II and III) includes the IMMUNE GLOBULINS which

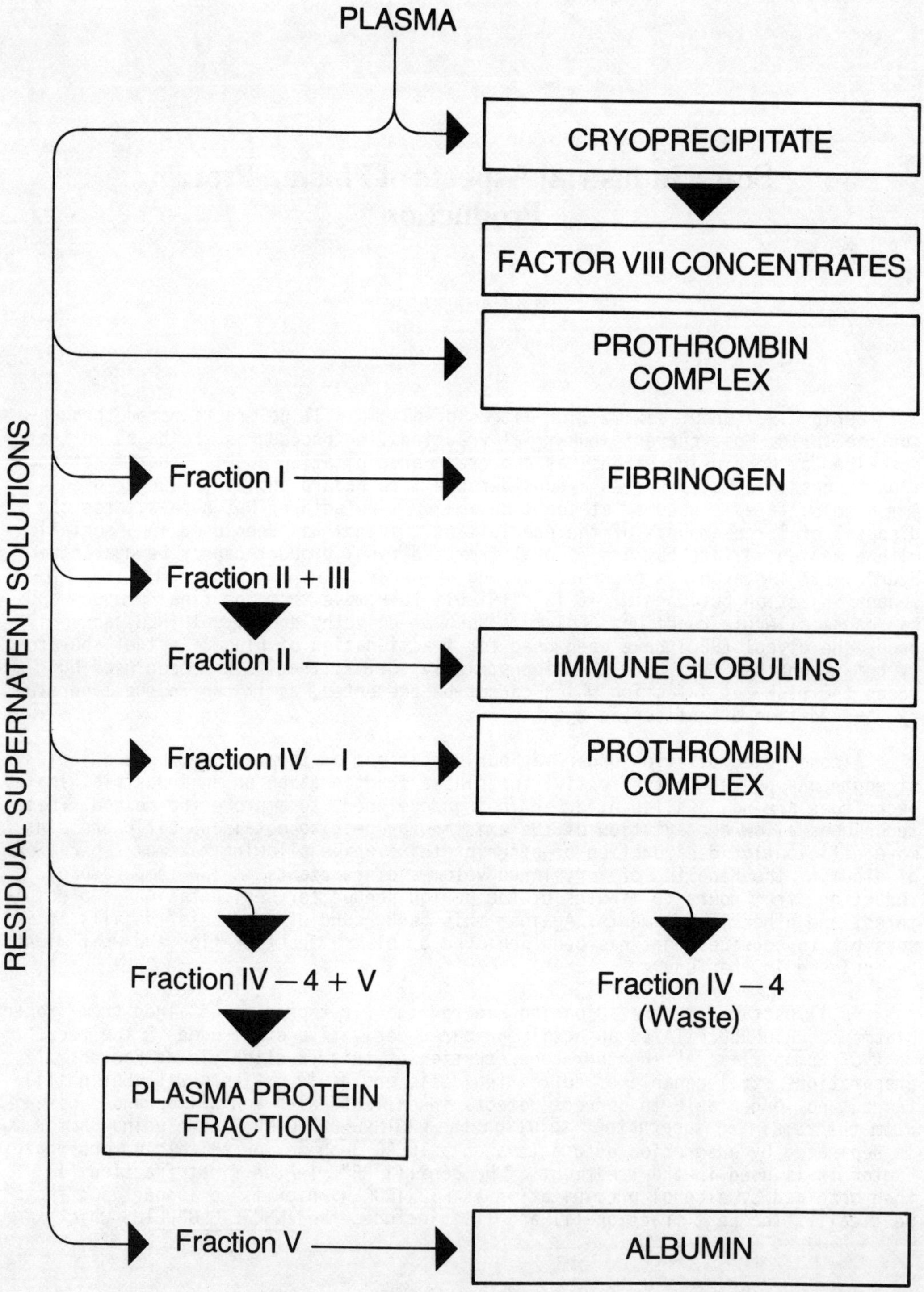
PLASMA
CRYOPRECIPITATE
FACTOR VIII CONCENTRATES
PROTHROMBIN COMPLEX
RESIDUAL SUPERNATENT SOLUTIONS
Fraction I
FIBRINOGEN
Fraction II + III
Fraction II
IMMUNE GLOBULINS
Fraction IV – I
PROTHROMBIN COMPLEX
Fraction IV – 4 + V
Fraction IV – 4 (Waste)
PLASMA PROTEIN FRACTION
Fraction V
ALBUMIN

require further precipitant fractionation for purification (II). If not removed by adsorption at an earlier phase, the prothrombin complex can be isolated from the next precipitate (IV-1). From the remaining supernatent solution it is then possible either to obtain PLASMA PROTEIN FRACTION. (IV-4 and V), containing more than 83% albumin, or a more highly purified preparation (more than 95-96%) of ALBUMIN (V) from which salt may have to be removed. Other fractions which have been obtained are THROMBIN used topically to control bleeding; FACTOR XIII, an amidolytic enzyme used to stabilize fibrin during wound healing; and PLASMINOGEN, now being used successfully in the treatment of hyaline membrane disease.

Trends in the future will depend upon improvements in existing techniques and products and on needs for individual fractions, some of which have not yet been isolated. The demands for albumin and plasma protein fraction, for example, could double in the next four or five years; they are currently used fo the treatment of shock, for nutritional purposes, and as a transport protein for drugs and toxic substances. In the field of immuno-therapy, there will be an increasing need for more specific preparations free of aggregates and having no anticomplementary activity. To obtain such preparations immune globulin fractions are being treated with enzymes such as pepsin or plasmin; with chemicals such as β propriolactone; or by filtration procedures to remove aggregates. The trouble is that these methods are either not entirely suitable or do not prevent reaggregation after removal of aggregates. In the future there will also be an increased demand for the elimination of infective agents from plasma products and for reduction of their side effects. At present the ability to exclude viruses is only as efficient as the sensitivities and specificities of the methods available for their detection in potential donors. Their elimination by inactivation is possible in some cases, such as albumin, but not in others where stability of the product is in jeopardy. There will be continued and possibly increased use of plasma fractions to supply the needs of deficient patients such as those requiring coagulation factors. Finally, needs which cannot now be satisfied could be met if techniques could be devised to separate and purify other plasma proteins. Thus α-1-antitrypsin might prove useful to treat some familiar forms of hepatitis in infancy and of emphysema in adults. Some forms of corneal ulcers are said to respond to treatment with serum α-2-macroglobulins. Anti-thrombin III might be needed as an alternative to heparin in the prevention or treatment of thrombosis. Ceruloplasmin, known to be deficient in Wilson's disease, might prove of use in diseases such as schizoprenia where metabolism of this protein is also abnormal. Haptoglobin, which binds hemoglobin to give a complex rapidly metabolized by the liver, might prove useful in the treatment of hemolytic anemia, a condition associated with haptoglobin depletion or absence. Hemoglobin itself might prove useful in place of intact red cells in cases of hemorrhagic shock under battle or other emergency conditions.

Progress is being made but much remains to be done. Each country or group of countries should assess its needs and assure its own supply of raw material, plasma. Since the problem is worldwide there is also a great need for exchange of information about resources and their development.

DISCUSSION

In discussion of the paper given by Dr.De Vreker the main topics considered were haptoglobins, hemoglobin, albumin and immune globulins.

Engler did not think that infusion of haptoglobin would prove useful in the treatment of haemolytic anemia. He pointed out, first, that the half-life of haptoglobin is about 3 days whereas that of the complex formed with hemoglobin is only 1 to 2 hours. Thus to correct the abnormally low haptoglobin levels seen in such patients, very large quantities would have to be given. Secondly, he felt that the phenotypes of the patients would have to be taken into consideration.

Hobbs pointed out the sequelae associated with repeated injection of hemoglobin, including renal complications and jaundice. He felt that use of hemoglobin under battle conditions might be warranted but not as an alternative under hospital conditions when red cells are available.

Hobbs also pointed out that amino acid infusions result in rapid urinary wastage and conversion to glucose without really conserving body proteins.Albumin, on the other hand, acts as a carrier of amino acids in the blood and can yield amino acids on degradation. He also emphasised that under extreme conditions of malnutrition absorption of food from the gut does not occur until infusions of albumin have been given to increase vital secretions into the gut. Amongst others, Peeters noted that albumin acts as an important carrier of fatty acids, an alternative source of energy in the malnourished. While not wishing to contradict the virtues of albumin, Dolkart emphasised that infused amino acids can only exert a nitrogen sparing action if they are given with adequate amounts of carbohydrate such as glucose, an assertion with which Hobbs did not entirely agree.

In response to a question from Intorp, De Vreker agreed that IgG3 immune globulins do readily aggregate and that their aggregation is favoured by calcium ions. It is not possible to prevent this, however, by adding chelating agents to commercial preparations, even if these immune globulins were responsible for aggregation. Their use would not be allowed in the U.S. Albumin has been used but plasmin may be more effective since it does degrade IgG3 molecules. Intorp suggested that solid phase chelating agents might prove useful to remove copper and calcium ions.

The Therapeutic Use of Human Immunoglobulins Selected on the Basis of Their Antibody Activity against Circulating Antigens

Pierre L. Masson

Brussels, Belgium

Recently, we have set up an agglutination inhibition test for detecting circulating immune complexes (8). By applying it to patients with Idiopathic Thrombocytopenic Purpura (ITP), we observed that the number of platelets was inversely proportional to the titre of immune complexes. In addition to immune complexes, we found viral antigens in the serum of most patients. This observation prompted us to undertake a clinical trial with human immunoglobulins (Ig) containing antibodies against viral antigens.

We have also applied the Ig treatment to children with recurrent infections of the upper respiratory tract. Seventy percent of these children have circulating antigens, free or in the form of immune complexes and presumably of infectious origin. In these patients we obtained a beneficial effect with the treatment provided that the injected Ig contained antibodies against the patient's circulating antigens (3). These observations could have practical consequences in paediatric practice but could also result in a new therapeutic approach to infectious diseases in general, or to some immune disorders which could be secondary to chronic infections.

Before describing the results of Ig treatment in ITP and in recurrent infections, it seems appropriate to describe briefly the agglutination inhibition test which is used for detecting not only immune complexes but also possible reactions of the Ig preparation with a patient's serum.

THE AGGLUTINATION INHIBITION TEST

The principle of this test rests on the ability of antigen-antibody complexes to react with rheumatoid factor or with Clq, a constituent of the first factor of complement. These two reagents have strong agglutinating activity toward particles coated with IgG. By competition with IgG present on the particles, the immune complexes inhibit agglutination.

The test is performed with two agglutinating reagents because rheumatoid factor and Clq have different specificities with respect to the Ig involved in the complexes and the size of the latter. In practice one volume of patient's serum is mixed on a dark plate with one volume of the suspension of IgG-coated polystyrene particles ("latex"), and one volume of rheumatoid serum or Clq. To obtain great sensitivity, the agglutinating reagents must be diluted as much as possible.

The inhibitory activity is expressed as the highest dilution of patient's serum still producing clear inhibition.

For selecting the Ig preparation for treatment, the patient's serum is first incubated with the Ig for about 30 min, and the inhibitory activity of the mixture is compared with those of the serum and the Ig preparation alone. The Ig batches which cause a significant increase of at least two dilution titres in the inhibition titre are chosen for use in treatment.

THE Ig TREATMENT OF ITP

The clinical trials with Ig were undertaken on the working hypothesis that circulating viral antigens are involved in the pathogenesis of thrombocytopenia. However, we could not exclude the possibility that their presence in the serum is due to immune depression resulting from treatment with prednisone or azathioprine. A beneficial effect of the Ig injections should, of course, be a convincing argument for the pathogenic role of viral infections.

So far, using the counter-electrophoresis technique, we have identified antigens from only three types of virus. Forty-two ITP sera were tested and of these 20 (48%) reacted positively to a convalescent anti-HBs antigen serum, 5 (12%) to a convalescent anti-Epstein-Barr virus serum, and 6 (14%) to horse or convalescent anti-adenovirus sera. Apparently, these circulating antigens were not constituents of immune complexes. In a study of two patients' sera we observed, after isolation of the complexes and their dissociation, that their antigen consisted of DNA. Whether this DNA originated from the tissues or from the viruses remains an open question.

Theoretically, these antigens could lead to destruction of platelets by any of three mechanisms. First, the antigens could be adsorbed on to the platelets as has been described for influenza virus (2). The damage to platelets should then be a consequence of the reaction between anti-viral antibodies and adsorbed antigens. Secondly, the viral infection could trigger auto-immune reactions against platelets. It is well established that destruction of platelets is related to the occurrence of a serum factor containing IgG (6), and several authors (5,7) believe that this factor represents auto-antibody. However, it has not been demonstrated that the IgG reacts via its Fab fragment with platelets and it is not excluded that the IgG containing factors of the ITP sera are immune complexes rather than auto-antibodies. Finally, immune complexes are known to be capable of agglutinating platelets. Such a reaction is even used for detecting immune complexes (12). So, the occurrence of circulating immune complexes in all ITP sera, and the reciprocal relationships between their titres and the count of platelet support the hypothesis that ITP is an immune complex disease, like other forms of thrombocytopenia such as acute post-infectious (11) and drug-induced immunologic thrombocytopenia (9,13).

With A. Lurhuma and M. Delire, we have treated 11 ITP patients with Ig. No change was observed in three, but in the other eight, an improvement or remission was observed concomitant with the Ig injections. So far, we have no statistical data proving that the favourable outcome was due to Ig treatment. However the changes in platelet count occurring in some patients were apparently related to the dosage of Ig and do suggest real therapeutic activity. In some cases the effect of Ig was transient. In others the improvement or remission persisted after stopping the injections but some patients required more persistent treatment.

Three typical cases will now be described:

Patient Du. This 62 year-old woman had had ITP for 25 years . The only treatment she received before the Ig injections was a regular dose of prednisone (10 mg/

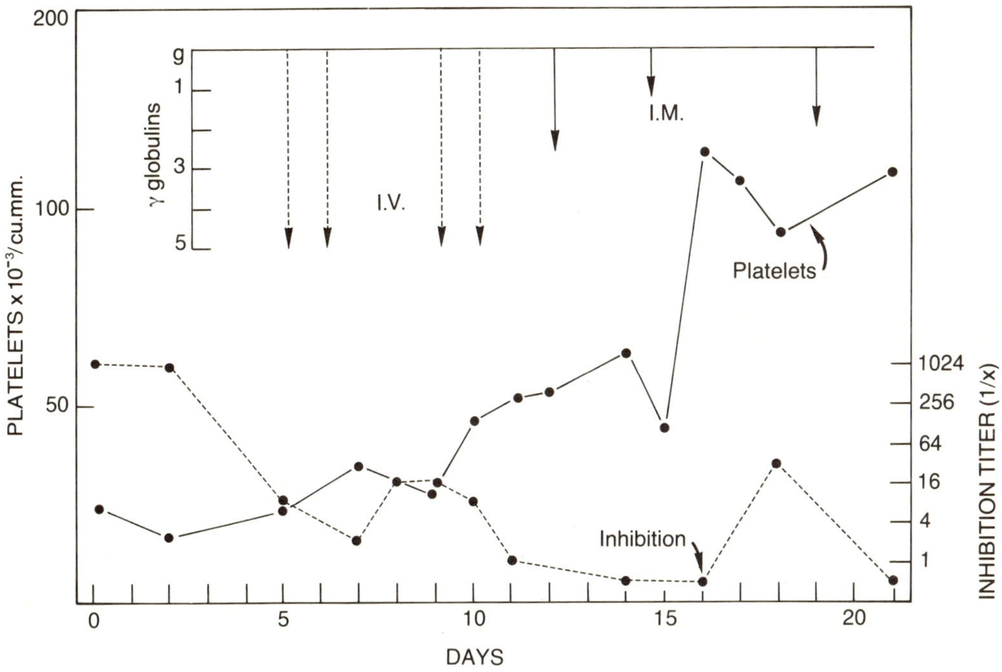

Figure 1. Responses of patient Du to repeated intravenous (IV) and intramuscular (IM) injections of Ig (g). Changes are shown for platelet count and inhibition of Clq by serum in the presence of the Ig preparation used for treatment over a period between June 9 and June 30, 1975.

day). Splenectomy was considered but rejected as platelet sequestration was diffuse. A temporal arteritis was diagnosed in 1973 by arterial biopsy. In June 1975 she was hospitalized for ecchymoses. Her platelet count was 20,000 per cu.mm. Hepatitis Bs antigen was found by counter-electrophoresis. Circulating immune complexes were detected by their reaction with rheumatoid factor (titre 1/32) and with Clq (titre 1/32).

The Ig treatment started with 4 infusions of 5 g of a plasmin-treated preparation (Veinoglobulines, Institut Mérieux, Lyon, France) in a week. The next week the patient received 3 intramuscular injections corresponding to a total of 5.4g. Both batches of Ig had strong antibody activity against the circulating antigen.

During the first week, a slow increase of platelet count was observed, followed, after the first intramuscular injection, by a rapid rise to 110,000 platelets per cu.mm (Figure 1). The inhibition titres toward Clq, measured in the presence of the preparation of Ig changed in a reciprocal way to the platelet count, suggesting progressive disappearance of the circulating antigen.

The prednisone treatment was continued during and after the Ig treatment because of the temporal arteritis. Two controls in 1976 gave platelet counts of 84,000 and 77,000 per cu.mm and no inhibition of Clq or rheumatoid factor. However, a slight agglutinating activity, presumably due to endogenous rheumatoid factor, was noted in these two controls. The patient claimed that treatment with Ig had decreased headaches caused by her temporal arteritis.

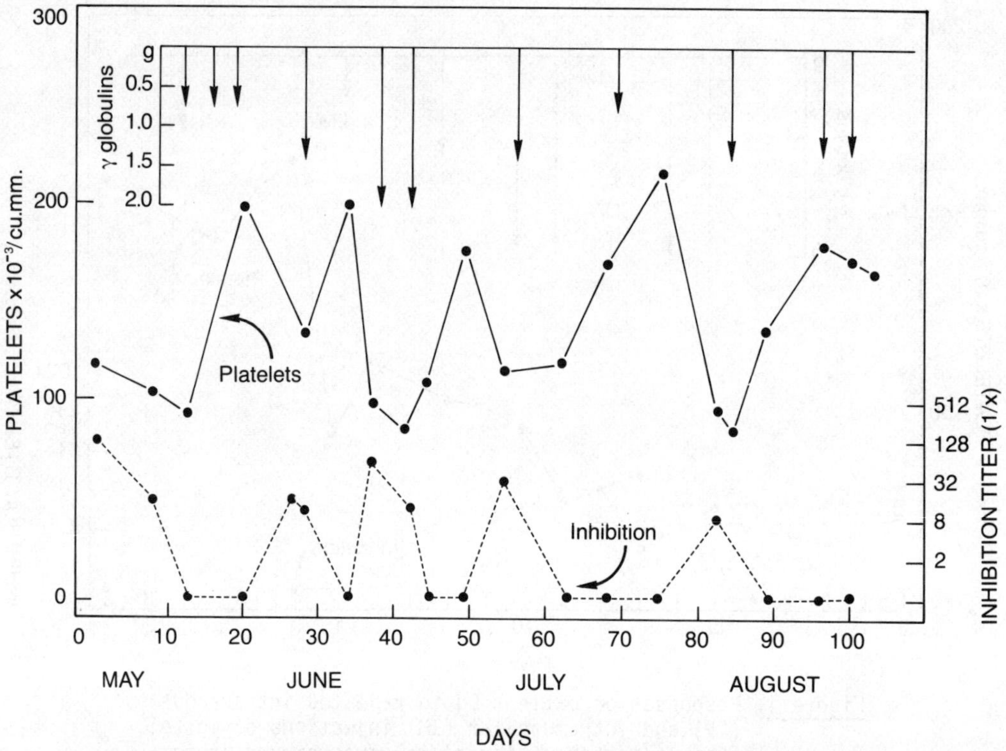

Figure 2. Responses of patient Ba during 100 days (May 21 to August 29, 1975) to repeated intramuscular injections of Ig (g). The symbols refer to measurements defined in Figure 1.

Patient Ba. This 55 year-old woman had had ITP since May 1973 with sequestration of platelets in the liver and spleen. In spite of high doses of prednisone (80 mg/day), the platelet count never exceeded 30,000 per cu.mm. In May 1975, azathioprine (150 mg/day) was added to prednisone whose dose was progressively reduced. After marked improvement with platelet counts exceeding 150,000 per cu.mm, a relapse occurred in January 1975, again requiring high doses of prednisone (100 mg/day).

In June 1975, the patient's serum was tested for immune complexes. Slight inhibitions of Clq (1/2) and of rheumatoid factor (1/2) were observed. Adenovirus antigens were detected by counter-electrophoresis. A batch of Ig was selected and injected intra-muscularly. The doses are shown in Figure 2 which also shows the evolution of platelet count and of inhibitory activity towards Clq in the presence of Ig. From June to August 1975, the number of platelets remained above 100,000 per cu.mm despite progressive decrease of prednisone dosage (40 mg/day in June, 35 mg/day in July, and 10 mg/day in August). During this period the platelet count oscillated regularly, increases being generally preceded by an injection of Ig. The level of circulating antigen also oscillated but in inverse relation to the number of platelets.

After August 1975, treatment was continued with weekly injections of 1.2 g of Ig; treatment with prednisone was suspended. In December 1975, after an acute respiratory tract infection, the patient relapsed in spite of increasing dosage of Ig.

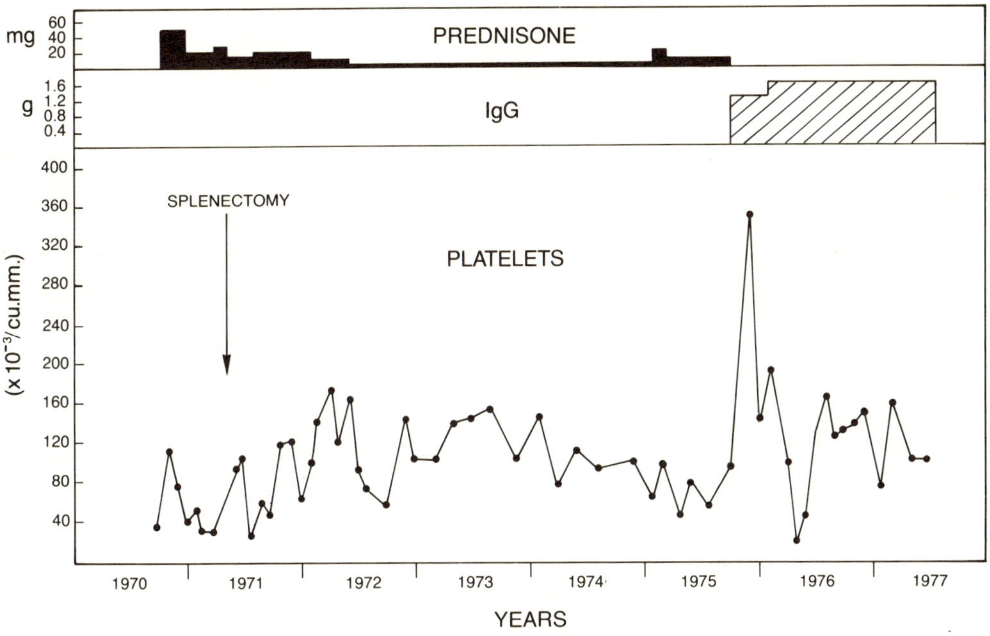

Figure 3. Responses of patient Ro between 1970 and 1977 to treatment by splenectomy and with prednisone (mg/day) and IgG (g/injection).

Patient Ro. (Figures 3 and 4). This 45 year-old man had had ITP since 1970. After splenectomy in 1971 and under prednisone treatment (5 to 20 mg/day), the platelet count, which was checked about every two months, varied between 20,000 and 160,000 /cu.mm. From January until August 1975, the platelets remained below 100,000 /cu.mm even after prednisone dosage had been increased to 20 mg/day for 1 month and 10 mg/day for 6 months (Figure 3).

In August 1975, adenovirus antigen was detected in the serum. A batch of Ig was selected and daily intramuscular injections of 1.2 g were started (Figure 4). The prednisone treatment was suspended. After 5 injections of 1.2 g and 6 injections of 1.6 g, the number of platelets peaked at 360,000 per cu.mm., and then with some intermediate lower peaks, went down to 25,000 per cu.mm. This decrease was concomitant with a reduction in the number of injections (2/month). In May 1976 weekly injections were therefore resumed. From May 1976 until September,1977, three reductions of Ig dosage were attempted. The first two were followed by relapses (below 100,000 per cu.mm) requiring readjustment of treatment. Since the third attempt in March 1977 the platelet counts have oscillated in the normal range (above 100,000 per cu.mm.).

Of course, these preliminary results cannot be considered as definitive proof of the therapeutic effect of Ig in ITP. Furthermore, if the Ig were really responsible for the increased platelet counts it remains to be demonstrated that improvement was due to antibody activity of the Ig injections and not to a non-specific effect of Ig. The IgG aggregates present in the preparation could, for example, activate complement, and this partial consumption of complement could then reduce platelet destruction. Clinical trials with Ig devoid of antibody activity on circulating antigen should now be carried out.

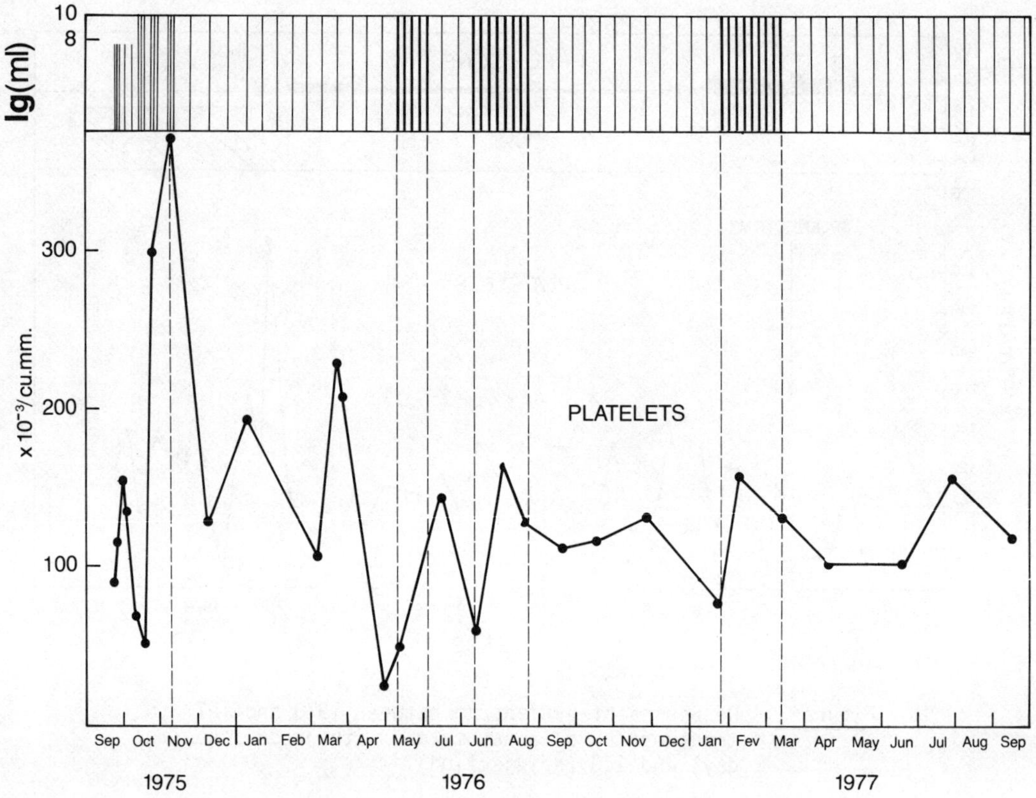

Figure 4. Effects produced between 1975 and 1977 by differing frequencies of injection of Ig (ml; 160 mg Ig/ml) upon platelet count of patient Ro.

THE Ig TREATMENT OF RECURRENT INFECTIONS

Recurrent upper respiratory tract infections present one of the most frustrating clinical problems facing pediatricians. There is some evidence that injection of Ig provides a useful form of treatment. However its efficacy has never been clearly proved and such treatment is indeed considered by some to be totally ineffective (10). The detection of circulating immune complexes in common infections of the upper respiratory tract gave us the idea that it might be possible to treat these patients effectively with Ig containing specific antibodies against the patient's circulating antigens, whether free or bound in immune complexes. This postulated therapeutic approach is supported by the results of an initial trial on 39 children (3) and has recently been confirmed in a second study of 67 children (4). These data will now be summarized and considered together.

The clinical trials consisted of injections of the same batch of Ig into all children in the study, of following their clinical course, and of correlating clinical and biological improvements with antibody activity against the circulating antigen of the injected preparation of Ig. The operator who performed the serological tests did not know the clinical data, and the clinicians were unaware of the results of laboratory tests. This study could be considered as double blind, the patients receiving the Ig without antibody activity constituting the control group. The children were aged 18 months to 6 years. All had had at least five in-

Table 1

REACTIONS OF PATIENTS SERA BEFORE TREATMENT WITH Ig (+)	SIGNIFICANT IMPROVEMENT FOLLOWING TREATMENT WITH Ig (*)
POSITIVE (n = 57)	39/57 (68%)
NEGATIVE (n = 40)	4/40 (10%)

Table 1. Responses of 97 patients to Treatment with Ig. Improvement was considered significant (*) when no more than one infectious episode was observed during five months and/or reversion towards normal was seen in the serum protein profile, circulating immune complexes or serum antigens. The correlation between reaction of patients' sera before treatment (+) and subsequent response to treatment was significant ($p < 0.001$).

fectious episodes (otitis media, pharyngitis, or tonsillitis) with fever of 38°C or more during the cold season (November to March) before the clinical trial. During November and December each patient received three intramuscular injections of 0.66 g of Ig of placental origin (Gamma 16, Institut Mérieux, Lyon, France) at 14 to 20 day intervals in the first study and at weekly intervals in the second. A single batch was used for all patients. Each child was then clinically examined at least once a month until March. The patients were also checked by laboratory tests, including determination of serum proteins (albumin, α1-antitrypsin, orosomucoid, haptoglobin, transferrin, C3 and C4 factors of complement, IgA, IgM and IgG) and of circulating immune complexes or antigens. The tests were performed on serum samples collected 48 hours before and 6 weeks after the first Ig injection. Before treatment most children (85%) had one or more abnormal laboratory tests. In 10 children a slight agglutinating activity was detected. It presumably corresponded to rheumatoid factor, which, as shown earlier (8), indicates the presence of circulating immune complexes.

Whatever the criteria used for assessing progress of patients (i.e. clinical outcome, normalization of the laboratory tests or both), a close correlation ($P < 0.001$) was established between the beneficial effects of Ig and the in vitro antibody activity of Ig against antigens present in pre-treatment sera of the patient (Table 1). In addition to the disappearance of circulating antigens or immune complexes and regression of the inflammatory reaction, the concentrations of IgA, IgM, and IgG decreased during treatment, especially in the group of patients with other signs of improvement. Statistically significant decreases of IgM and IgG (Table 2) were observed only in the population of children who, before treatment, had circulating antigens reacting with antibodies in the Ig preparation.

The half-life of IgG being about 20 days, the prolonged effect of the Ig treatment for more than 3 to 5 months after the last injection was unexpected. As immune complexes are suspected of interfering with cellular immunity (1,14) it is possible that elimination of immune complexes by Ig could "unblock" cellular immunity and allow the children to mount their own immune response. For testing this hypothesis, we performed skin tests with candidine and streptokinase-streptodorna-

Table 2

GROUPS OF PATIENTS	DECREASE * IN SERUM IgG LEVEL (MEAN ± SD)
PATIENTS WHO AFTER TREATMENT SHOWED:	
(i) IMPROVEMENT (n = 25)	5.9 ± 2.4**
(ii) NO IMPROVEMENT (n = 33)	1.8 ± 3.7
PATIENTS WHOSE SERA BEFORE TREATMENT:	
(i) REACTED WITH Ig (n = 33)	6.3 ± 2.8**
(ii) DID NOT REACT WITH Ig (n = 25)	0.4 ± 3.9

Table 2. Decreases in serum IgG levels of 58 patients treated with Ig. Criteria for improvement induced by treatment are defined under Table 1. The IgG levels before and after treatment were originally expressed as percentages of the normal absolute value for adults.The decreases shown here (*) refer to mean differences (± SD) between these percentage values. Significant decreases ($p < 0.05$) induced by treatment are shown.(**)

se (Varidase) before and after treatment. If the children had an impairment of their cellular immunity, a low proportion of positive skin tests should have been observed before treatment. Referring to the literature, our results with candidine before treatment did not differ significantly, whereas for Varidase the proportion (11%) was clearly lower than the values (46-47%) reported by others (15). After treatment, the positive tests for Varidase reached 41% . The six week-interval can hardly account for this increased proportion of positive tests. Probably this evolution was related to the favourable clinical outcome. However, the correlation between clinical and biological improvement and the fact that the Varidase test became positive was hardly significant ($0.1 < P > 0.05$).

The batch of Ig used for the clinical trials gave a positive antibody reaction in 55% of the sera. Three other batches of placental Ig, which were tested only on some pre-treatment patient sera, gave positive reactions in 50%, 44% and 43%, respectively. We have also observed that sera with circulating antigens reacting with none of the Ig batches were scarce (2 out of 36); most sera reacted with at least two of the tested batches of Ig. Therefore, it seems that most antigens are quite common. However, we do not yet know the nature of the bacteria or viruses which, presumably, are the sources of these antigens. The children which were not improved by the Ig should now be treated with selected batches. Then it will be possible to see whether they resisted the first injections because of absence of antibody in the preparation or for some other unknown reason.

Acknowledgment. We thank Dr. A. Leek for corrections. This work was supported by the Cancer Research Fund of the Caisse Générale d'Epargne et de Retraite,Brussels.

REFERENCES

1. Baldwin, R.W., Price, M.R. and Robins, R.A., Blocking of lymphocyte-mediated cytotoxicity for rat hepatoma cells by tumor-specific antigen-antibody complexes. Nature-New Biol. 238, 185 (1972)

2. Danon, D., Jerushalmy, Z. and De Vries, A. Incorporation of influenza virus in human blood platelets in vitro. Virology 9, 719 (1959)

3. Delire, M. and Masson, P.L. The detection of circulating immune complexes in children with recurrent infections and their treatment with human immunoglobulins. Clin.Exp.Immunol. (in press).

4. Delire, M.,Petit, B., Fiasse, L. and Masson, P.L. Correlation between the therapeutic efficacy of human immunoglobulins and their in vitro antibody activity on circulating antigens in children with recurrent infections (submitted).

5. Dixon, R.H.and Rosse, W.F. Platelet antibody in autoimmune thrombocytopenia. Brit.J.Haematol.31, 129 (1975).

6. Harrington, W.J., Minnich, V., Hollingsworth, J.W. and Moore, C.V. Demonstration of a thrombocytopenic factor in the blood of patients with thrombocytopenic purpura. J.Lab.Clin.Med. 38, 1 (1951).

7. Karpatkin, S. and Siskind, G.W. In vitro detection of platelet antibody in patients with idiopathic thrombocytopenic purpura and systemic lupus erythematosus. Blood 33, 795 (1969).

8. Lurhuma, A.Z., Cambiaso, C.L., Masson, P.L. and Heremans, J.F. Detection of circulating antigen-antibody complexes by their inhibitory effect on the agglutination of IgG-coated particles by rheumatoid factor or Clq. Clin.Exp.Immunol. 25, 212 (1976).

9. Miescher, P. and Miescher, R. Die Sedormid-Anaphylaxis. Schweiz Med.Wschr.82, 1279 (1952).

10. Miller, M.E. Use and abuses of plasma therapy in the patient with recurrent infections. J.Allergy Clin. Immunol. 51, 45 (1973)

11. Myllylä, G., Vaheri, A., Vesikari, T. and Penttinen, K. Interaction between human blood platelets, viruses, and antibodies. IV. Post rubella thrombocytopenic purpura and platelet aggregation by rubella antigen-antibody interaction. Clin.Exp.Immunol. 4, 323 (1969).

12. Penttinen, K., Vaheri, A. and Myllylä, G. Detection and characterization of immune complexes by the platelet aggregation test. I. Complexes formed in vitro Clin. Exp. Immunol. 8, 389 (1971).

13. Shulman, N.R. A mechanism of cell destruction in individuals sensitized to foreign antigens and its implications in autoimmunity. Ann.Intern.Med. 60,506 (1964).

14. Sjögren, H.O., Hellström, I., Bansal, S.C. and Hellström, K.E. Suggestive evidence that the"blocking antibodies" of tumour-bearing individuals may be antigen-antibody complexes. Proc.Nat.Acad.Sci.68, 1372 (1971).

15. Steele, R.W. Suttle, D.E., Le Master, P.C., Patterson, F.D. and Canales, L. Screening of all mediated immunity in children. Amer.J.Dis.Child. 130,1218 (1976).

DISCUSSION

Discussion of Professor Masson's paper centred around possible methods for treating diseases associated with circulating antibodies. Treatment could be directed towards alleviation of symptoms or towards removal or suppression of the basic cause of their appearance. As an example, Masson pointed out that diabetes is considered by some to be an autoimmune disease. The stimulus for its appearance could be a virus and the responsible antigen a component of the damaged β-cells such as insulin. Susceptible persons could be identified,at an early age, possibly by virtue of their HLA grouping. The appearance of antibodies causing the diabetic syndrome could then be prevented in some practical manner. De Vreker described the appearance in the blood of some hemophilic patients of inhibitors which render them resistant to treatment with Factor VIII. When very large doses of Factor VIII are given to such resistant patients, bleeding episodes are reduced in number and the inhibitors are said ultimately to disappear from the blood. Ballieux reported the results of studies which he had carried out in vitro and in which he was able to suppress antibody production by human lymphocytes. He first showed that if lymphocytes are incubated for 5 days in vitro they can then be induced to produce antibodies to such antigens such as sheep red blood cells or ovalbumin. If,however, they are first exposed for a day to high concentrations of an antigen and are then incubated for five days in its absence, those lymphocytes cannot then be stimulated to produce antibodies to that antigen. Their ability to produce antibodies is suppressed.(1) It thus emerged that antibody production could be suppressed by two methods. The antibody producing human or animal subject could be exposed in vivo to very high doses of the antigen. Alternatively, lymphocytes from the affected subject could be induced to have a suppressive effect on antibody production during incubation in vitro and might then be infused into the donor to exert the same effect in vivo. In either case production of antibodies responsible for the disease could be prevented or arrested. Practical difficulties still remain to be solved before such methods could be tried in the patient. The antigens responsible for many diseases have yet to be identified and actions of suppressed lymphocytes remain to be assessed in vivo.

REFERENCE

1. Uyte De Haag, F., Heynen, C.J. and Ballieux, R.E. Induction of antigen-specific human suppressor T-lymphocytes in vitro. Nature 271, 556 (1978).

Standardisation of Protein Assays

John R. Hobbs

London, England

Standardisation is an ongoing process, taking continuous account of advancing methodology and the improved preparation of reference standards, yet continuing also to monitor the stability of standard materials that have been prepared. The process should also take account of a hierarchy of levels of acceptance. Definitive standards and methods are as close to the absolute truth as is possible at any moment in time, and on the whole are very impractical and very expensive. Reference standards and methods are those applicable in a wide variety of expert laboratories but may again be impractical for routine analyses. Recommended standards and methods are those which will give an acceptable result in a working laboratory. Finally, while this is but a very brief summary of many documents from the IFCC, WHO and IUIS which discuss the philosophy of standardisation, a final criterion that I insist on is that any recommended method or standard should have been well tried in the field before it is accepted. I just briefly wish to consider work that has been done with albumin, IgG, IgA and IgM, and to mention the problems associated with C3.

ALBUMIN

Following a review of albumin methodology and a field trial of albumin standardisation both in normal and abnormal samples (3), it became obvious that immunochemical methods for estimating albumin were the best. Of these, the one most easily taken up in other laboratories to yield a precision of plus or minus 0.6% in the measurement of albumin in normal serum, was the Laurell rocket method. This method was also best with regard to abnormal sera. Both the rocket and the Mancini methods had the advantage that any impurities in anti-albumin do not register in the visible precipitin lines, but rather as ghost rings or peaks clearly distinguishable from those on which the reading is made. For nephelometry it is essential that no impurities are present as these will add to the turbidometric reading. There is furthermore the problem of complexing of albumin to other substances such as kappa light chains, IgA, myeloma proteins, etc., which have to be considered when dealing with abnormal samples. For this reason the IFCC Expert Panel on Proteins has recommended the Laurell rocket method as the method for calibration when comparing standard materials. For that purpose it does possess a reference anti-albumin which is known to give reliable, clean rocket peaks. For immunochemical methods which involve migration or complex formation, the size of the albumin appears to be critical.

In normal and in most abnormal sera, albumin exists almost entirely in monomer form. In contrast almost all highly purified dried human serum albumin powders contain polymers or form them when the solution is reconstituted. Among 18 such powders examined by the Expert Panel on Proteins the majority contained 10% dimer. However, it has recently been claimed that acetone drying can greatly reduce their amount (4). A further anomaly was found in that it was possible to obtain a constant UV absorption at 280 nm. Thus if a solution of albumin is read, dried to constant weight after dialysis against a variety of solutions, and then reconstituted to its original exact volume, a different UV reading is often obtained. We therefore felt it was unsatisfactory to ascribe to an albumin powder a projected UV value. It was also not acceptable to assume that human albumin contains 16% nitrogen and to standardise it by Kjeldahl.

All of this was taken into account when making a specification for a human serum albumin reference standard which as yet no firm has considered producing. Among the preparations examined at that time was an albumin solution prepared by electrophoresis. This met most of the requirements of our specification: it was almost wholly monomeric and was 99.6% pure human albumin on careful immunoelectrophoretic checking. It was therefore adopted as a working standard and its mass value was taken after the material had been dialysed against ammonium formate and freeze dried to constant weight with careful checking of its conductivity and water content. Against this standard, the IFCC standard serum 74/1 was measured in no less than 12 different countries by the above recommended procedures. The means from those twelve different countries showed a total variation of 39.8 to 40.7 g/l, with an overall mean of 40.3 g/l the value ascribed to 74/1. Unfortunately the working standard of human albumin has all been used, and no reference material has since met the required specification. Even triply-crystallised human serum albumin forms 11% polymers on solution. Dr. Th. Peters of the USA is experimenting with the blocking of isolated monomer to try and prevent reaggregation in solution. Meanwhile, I personally can only recommend the use of IFCC 74/1 for which we have a very precise assay of albumin content; a recent check showed that in the "wet" standard, 74/1, the albumin was still 99% in monomer form.

IgG, IgA AND IgM

There does exist for serum immunoglobulin a WHO international standard which is distributed in the UK as 67/99 and which shows some variance in content with regard to dry weight. Personally, I have found that if 10 ampoules are each reconstituted by addition of 1 ml of distilled water and then pooled the variance between ampoules is ironed out and the content can then be assumed to be 96.2 IU/ml. I would hasten to add that this is not the way recommended by the WHO for using the standard. They in fact, hope that users will weigh the vial before and after its contents have been dissolved and removed so that any correction can be made for any variance observed in the original dry weight within that ampoule. The reconstituted serum is turbid and unsuitable for nephelometry, except where a laser is read at an angle or where it is used at high dilution. For the WHO standard there are also agreed milligram equivalents (1).

Five protein Reference Units in the United Kingdom undertook a study of methodology in comparing the WHO standard against IFCC 74/1 and this will shortly be published (5). Satisfactory parallel line assays were obtained by most methods but not for IgM by nephelometry. Since, however, the WHO standard was simply designed and itself calibrated by Mancini, it was from these results that the calibration was chosen. Furthermore, it was discovered on complete analysis of the raw data that, when the Mancini readings were computed rather than manually drawn, both the coefficients of variation and the standard errors of the estimates were markedly reduced. (CVs between five centres, between batches, show overall spreads of 2.8 to 5.8%). As a result of this study we have been able to assign values for immunoglobulins in 74/1 of IgA, 102 IU ml or 1.45 g/l : IgG, 108 IU ml or 8.68 g/l: and IgM, 146 IU ml or 1.24 g/l. The IFCC 74/1 solution is suitable for nephelometry. For IgG there was no method-specific variance outside the variance of the assays, but for IgA there was a consistent trend to obtain high results by both Laurell rocket (2) and automated immune precipitation methods as compared to the Mancini method. For IgM there was very close agreement between the formulated rockets and Mancini values.

It is therefore possible to measure an unknown for its content of immunoglobulins either against WHO 67/99 using Mancini only, or against IFCC 74/1 using other methods, with the above qualifications. In absolute terms there are at the moment no satisfactory pure immunoglobulin standards to assign more accurate concentration than the above standards. However, in the meanwhile we can at least refer all unknowns to the original WHO preparation, and this will at least make comparison possible between different countries and different laboratories. In the continuing process of standardisation it is hoped that at some time in the future better absolute values will be ascribed to the existing standards.

COMPLEMENT-C

An IUIS Sub-Committee on Complement Standards has been considering the problems for some four years, and has not yet produced a standard material. A parallel sub-committee for a serum protein standard has completed its Phase I studies and is recommending a freeze-dried human serum pool (Freon-treated) for acceptance as a standard. This material, stored from 4 to -70°C, shows no significant conversion of C3 after 6 months. A batch of similar material is to be studied by the Complement Sub-Committee to see if it could be adopted as a complement standard. It is worth giving the warning that IFCC 74/1 showed no significant conversion of C3 for two years, but then suddenly developed 30% conversion, even at -70°C, in the third year in an unpredictable manner by the usual thermal stability studies. Thus, while initially 74/1 gave a very clean rocket peak in C3 estimation it now after three years produces a small tail at the top of the peak and in my opinion this invalidates its use as a reference standard for the rocket measurement of C3. It remains to be seen whether the same problems will occur with the new proposed standard; they do not exist at present. In the absence of an absolute reference of purified C3, it is not at present possible to ascribe mass value to any working serum and the IUIS proposes to assign a unitage to its new standard. If its C3 content remains in native form, it will at least provide a reference material in the next year or two, until, we hope, the continuing process of standardisation produces better complement standards.

CONCLUSION

At present there are no definitive standards for albumin, IgG, IgM or C3. IFCC 74/1 seems to represent a suitable reference material for albumin, IgG,IgA, IgM, when recommended methods and reliable antisera have been tested in the field. WHO 67/99 represents a reference material for IgG, IgA and IgM but only when the Mancini method of calibration is used and used carefully. It is hoped a suitable C3 material will become available shortly.

REFERENCES

1. Humphrey, J.H. and Batty, I. International Reference preparation for human serum IgG, IgA and IgM. Clin.Exp.Immunol. 17,708 (1974).

2. Slater, L. IgG, IgA and IgM by formylated rocket immunoelectrophoresis, Ann. Clin.Bioch. 12,19 (1975).

3. Slater, L. Carter, P.M. and Hobbs, J.R. Measurement of albumin in the sera of patients. Ann.Clin.Bioch. 12,33 (1975).

4. Solli, N.J. and Bertolini, M.J. Polymer distribution in human serum albumin powders prepared by lyophilization or acetone drying. Vox Sang. 32,239 (1977).

5. Whicher, J.T., Hunt, J., Perry, D.E., Hobbs, J.R., Fifield, R., Keyser, J., Kohn, J.,Riches, P., Smith, A.M., Thompson, R.A., Milford Ward, A., and White, P. Method-specific variations in the calibration of a new immunoglobulin standard suitable for use in nephelometric techniques. Clin.Chem. 24,531(1978).

DISCUSSION

The problems associated with albumin monomers were confirmed by Peeters. In his experience a pure albumin solution separates into a broad area of fractions in an isotachophoretic column and this is the expression of the fatty acid load carried by albumin. After delipidation the albumin monomers show only one single protein peak but when fatty acids are added in amounts from one to six molecules per molecule of albumin a multitude of peaks reappears all with slightly different mobilities. The albumin thus gives the impression of being a heterogeneous substance. He proposes to prepare albumin solutions in which the amounts of fatty acid and salt are precisely determined. Although Hobbs considered that reference solutions are no substitute for dry standards, Peeters believed his proposal remains valid for preparing adequate dry standards. The weight of the stabilizing molecules,namely fatty acids and salts,can be taken into account when calculating the weight of the protein standard. This would ensure stability and reproducibility on solution after dry storage.

The problems associated with immunoglobulins are also very complex. Hobbs mentioned that the primary IgA standard prepared by WHO had been checked by about 40 different laboratories in order to establish a so called WHO standard for IgA. However, the data obtained by those laboratories were scattered and the IgA standard value was nothing more than the average of the 40 estimates obtained in 40 different laboratories. When preparing dilutions of a commercial preparation the curves do not overlap with the standard dilutions and for this reason a simple correction factor is not sufficient to convert found values into WHO units. The origin of the so called standard IgA immunoglobulin may be one of the causes for this discrepency. Starting from purified myeloma monomers Hobbs and Heremans prepared polyclonal IgA and were able to find coinciding values.

Ballieux made an important suggestion. It is not enough to compare milligrams. What actually counts is biological activity. Just as when one has to measure the effect of extracorporeal circulation in open heart surgery, so one has to measure functional effects on the immune response, cellular or humoral. The dilution effect is easy to follow but how can we measure biological damage done to proteins. Precipitation and nephelometry do not solve this aspect of the problem.

Serrera emphasized that choice of an analytical laboratory method could very well depend upon the circumstances of the person making that choice. He could be working in a small provincial hospital, in a large regional or national center,or in an institution devoted solely to research. He might wish to establish a diagnosis or to provide evidence for a given prognosis. In this case he could use any of many screening techniques which are simple, widely used and well understood. He might wish to study some pathological aspect of a given specific protein for which more specific methods are available. Some have been automated and lend themselves well to clinical studies because the results are amenable to computerization and mathmatical analysis, factors of increasing importance in clinical laboratories. He might also need to detect abnormal proteins whose presence, even in minimal quantities, would be of great diagnostic value. In this instance, the specificity and sensitivity of a method would be more important than its precision. Finally there could be need for a method which provides technical information of no immediate practical value but which could later become important. Where such research is carried out the techniques could reach a degree of sophistication and complexity seldom necessary in other centres. The choice of a suitable method could also be influenced by financial considerations which in turn could affect the nature of equipment and the quality of technical assistance available in a laboratory. But there is still one other factor to consider. Frequently, and especially in countries such as Spain, there is insufficient information available to carry out required technical procedures. Progress in science is not solely due to new discoveries. It is also measured by the manner in which such new information is spread to those capable of using it. I believe that there is a need for better dissemination of information about plasmaproteins and perhaps the pharmaceutical industry could help. Hobbs agreed. Technical methods devised for use in hospitals should be practical and economical. Means should be found, as they are in some centres in the U.K., for training technicians. In requesting assistance for such training, however, the needs of the trainee should be clearly defined. Dolkart agreed and pointed out that industrial concerns do help by producing simple descriptions of reliable methods placed on the market. In addition, however, there is a need for instruction in the interpretation of data obtained with the various methods. In a final comment, Serrera felt that if help were given to improve laboratory practice, potential for research would ultimately appear in laboratories where none is now done.

Phenotypes and Immunological Estimation of Haptoglobin

Robert Engler

Paris, France

The production of monospecific antibodies to human haptoglobin (Hp) enables us to assay this protein by immunological methods. Two allelomorphic genes Hp1, and Hp2, allow for the existence of three phenotypes Hp1.1, Hp2.1 and Hp2.2. In the French population the distribution for the Hp1.1 phenotype is 14%, for Hp2.1. is 47% and for Hp2.2. is 38%. The problem which this poses is whether assay of Hp/anti Hp complexes in the patient is dependent on the phenotype of his haptoglobin.

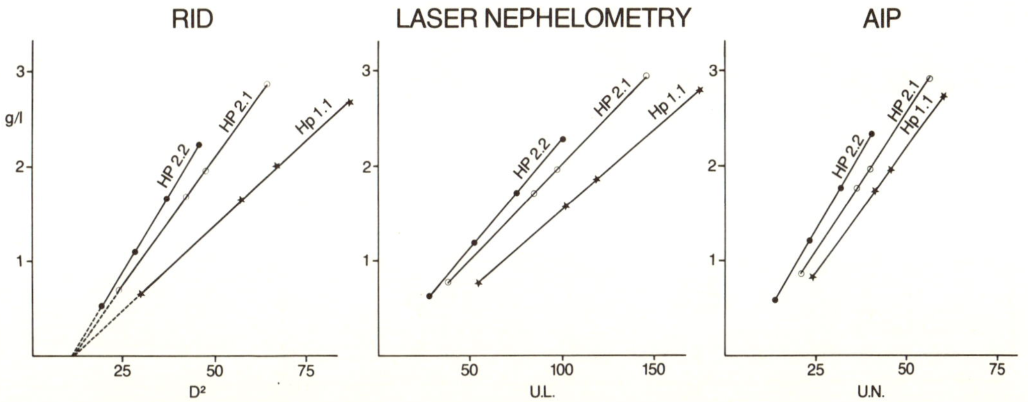

Figure 1. Experimental observations obtained by Radial Immunodiffusion (RID) laser nephelometry and Immunonephelometry (AIP) using solutions of pure haptoglobin of the three phenotypes (Hp1.1, Hp2.1 and Hp2.2.) in concentrations from 0 to 3 g/l (ordinate). The units shown on the abscissae are the square of the diameter of precipitate obtained by RID (D^2), and arbitrary units (UL and UN) measured by laser and immunophephelometry.

	R.I.D	LASER N.	A.I.P.
HP 1-1	1.5	1.5	1.5
HP 2-1	2.3	1.9	1.8
Hp 2-2	2.8	2.1	1.9
POOL serum	2.5	1.9	1.8

Table I. This shows the concentrations (g/l) of haptoglobin phenotypes Hp2.1 and Hp2.2. equivalent to that of a solution containing Hp1.1 in a concentration of 1.5g/l; these were calculated from data shown in Figure 1. Also shown is the equivalent for a pool of serum containing phenotypes in the proportions found in the French population.

In a preliminary study attempting to answer this question, we have isolated haptoglobins of all three phenotypes from ascitic fluid. Using known concentrations of the pure proteins, as measured by spectophotometric absorption at a wave-length of 280 nm (μg/l = 1.2), we have assayed them by three techniques - by radial immunodiffusion, by immunonephelometry (Technicon) and by Laser Nephelometry (Hyland).. The different values were then compared as functions of phenotypes.

MATERIALS AND METHODS

Starting with exudative ascitic fluid, the phenotypes were determined by a mathod perfected in this laboratory (1). The haptoglobins were prepared by ion exchange on DEAE-cellulose A50, followed by gel filtration chromatography (Ultrogel AC 44). The criteria for determination of purity were electrophoresis on polyacrylamide gel and immunoelectrophoresis with an immune-serum directed against all serum proteins.

RESULTS

The results obtained with solutions of the three pure phenotypes Hp.1, HP2.1. and Hp2.2. by the three methods of immunoassay are shown in Figure 1. At a concentration of 1.5 g/L for Hpl.1, the equivalent measured concentrations for phenotypes Hp2.1 and Hp2.2. derived from results in Figure 1 are shown in Table I. It is now possible to calculate a theoretical concentration of haptoglobin in a pool of serum containing the various phenotypes. In the case of a pool containing phenotypes in proportion to their distribution in the French population (see above), the value would be:

$$(2.3\ g/l \times 0.48) + (2.8\ g/l \times 0.38) + (1.5\ g/l \times 0.14) = 2.5\ g/l$$

Whichever immunochemical method is employed, the estimate of haptoglobin depends on the phenotype, the most varied results being obtained with radial immunodiffusion. However, for levels obtained in the zone of antibody excess, as with laser nephelometry and immunonephelometry (AIP), the values are very similar for Hp2.1, Hp2.2 and the pooled serum. For the estimation of haptoglobin in serum, two references might be used:

a. Using Hp2.1 for reference. To serum free of haptoglobulin from a subject with intravascular hemolysis is added a known concentration (3.0 g/l) of the phenotype Hp2.1. Using this solution for reference, and either of the techniques carried out in the liquid phase, only small correction factors would have to be applied in assays of the other phenotypes. The correction factors for Hpl.1. and Hp2.2. by laser nephelometry would be 0.83 and 1.08 and by immunonephelometry, 0.80 and 1.10. For clinical purposes, the phenotype present in the assay sample would therefore have little effect on the result of the assay and need not be considered. However, the correction coefficients for estimates made by immunodiffusion are 0.6 for HPl.1. and 1.2 for Hp2.2. Estimates made by this method could therefore be grossly inaccurate if the phenotype in the serum were not known.

b. Using pooled serum for reference. The values obtained using pooled serum for reference being the same as those using Hp2.1., one can apply the same arguments as those above. In defining the value for the pool as normal, the results can be expressed with reference to this value. Unfortunately in the case of an inflammatory reaction, the sera must be diluted so that the haptoglobin concentration falls within the range of assay.

CONCLUSIONS

An isolated estimate of serum haptoglobin provides the clinician with information on which he can act if the value is elevated (3 g/l) or very low (0.25g/l). The first suggests an acute inflammatory reaction and the second, where the value is low, suggest intravascular hemolysis. In these two instances the effect of phenotypes can be ignored. For sub-normal or moderately elevated levels of haptoglobin, determination of the phenotype seems to us of secondary importance with respect to the range of values for haptoglobin found in normal subjects. These values range between 0.6 g/l and 1.8 g/l. Beyond doubt an isolated estimate of haptoglobin is difficult to interpret. The ideal would be to determine in every person the normal basic level of haptoglobin (two estimates at intervals of two months in the case of the healthy subject) and, if possible, the phenotype. Since concentration of haptoglobin is remarkably constant in a person who has no inflammatory reaction, no intravascular hemolysis and no hepatic insufficiency, interpretation of slightly elevated values would take on clinical significance only if a patient's basic value were known.

REFERENCE

1. Engler, R., Rondeau, Y., Pointis, J. and Jayle, M.F. Activités péroxydatiques des combinaisons hémoglobiniques des trois phénotypes de l'haptoglobine. Clin. Chim.Acta. 47, 149 (1973).

DISCUSSION

In response to questions from Leyssens and Hobbs, Engler observed that he had used commercial antisera and antisera to Hp2.1 produced in his own rabbits. His own serum had given consistent results but with antisera from different companies he had obtained very variable estimates. More important, however, was the need for a reliable standard serum for reference; using a variety of currently available standards widely differing estimates are obtained by the same assay method.

Advantages of Small Angle Light Scattering Measurement in Immunonephelometry

Gregory J. Buffone and Susan A. Lewis

Washington, U.S.A.

The theoretical advantages of small angle (<90°) measurement of light scattering are well documented (1,2). At present no data are available to show the practical advantages of such measurements over light scattering at 90° under similar assay conditions. We present data to show the practical advantages of small angle measurement and compare results from instruments which measure light scattering at 90° and 31° relative to the sample position. The advantages and disadvantages of using undiluted serum specimens for this type of immunochemical assay are also presented.

METHODS AND MATERIALS

Antisera. Antihuman IgG, IgA, IgM and C3 were purchased from Atlantic Antibodies (Anderson Rd., Westbrook, ME 04092). Antihuman IgG was also obtained from Meloy Laboratories (6715 Electronic Dr., Springfield, VA 22151) and Hyland Laboratories (3300 Hyland Ave., Costa Mesa, CA 92626). Working antiserum dilutions were prepared in 40 g/liter polyethylene glycol, 0.15 mol/liter sodium chloride. Solutions of antiserum were left to stand 30 min. at room temperature and then filtered with a 0.45 μm filter (Millipore Corp., Bedford, MA 01730).

Calibration Serum. An assayed serum pool was obtained from Atlantic Antibodies (Lot RSC n°47). Assigned values for IgG, IgM, IgA and C3 were respectively 8.50, 1.14, 1.15 and 1.05 g/liter. Calibrators were diluted in 0.15 mol/liter NaCl for all experiments.

Nephelometer. Light scattering measurements were made using a commercial nephelometer (Hyland Laboratories). The angle of measurement is 31° relative to the sample position. All light scattering readings were made within 30 min. after initiation of a reaction, and are expressed in units of "relative light scattering" (% RLS) recommended by the manufacturers.

Results.

Assay performance was evaluated on the basis of slope, linearity and working analytical range of each assay. The working analytical range is defined as the range of concentration of protein antigen which can be measured in antibody excess with a relative precision of 5-10%. The methods considered were those for estimation of IgG, IgA, IgM and C3.

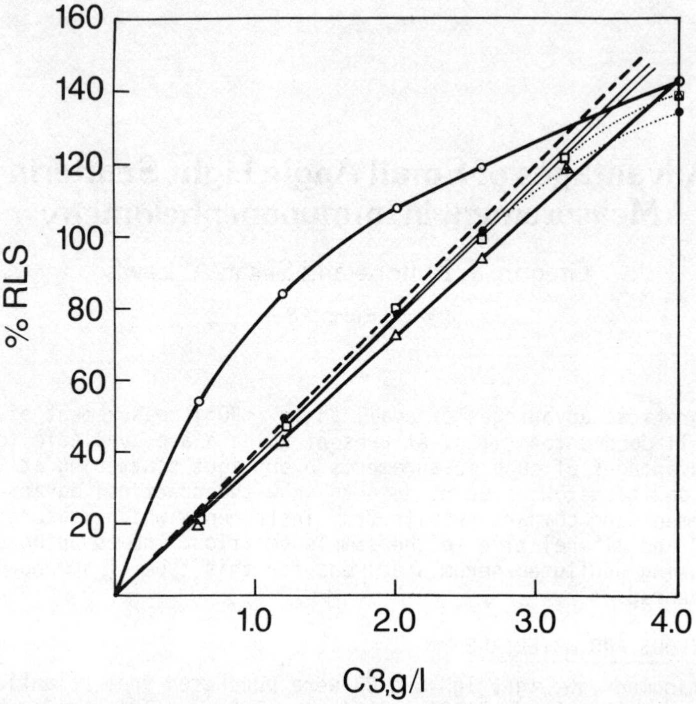

Figure 1. Light scattering (%RLS) after reaction between C3 (g/l) and antibody (Ab). The antibody (1:80) was allowed to react with undiluted serum (2μl; open circles); or, at dilutions of 1:80 (triangles), 1:200 (squares) and 1:800 (closed circles) with pre-diluted (1:100) serum.

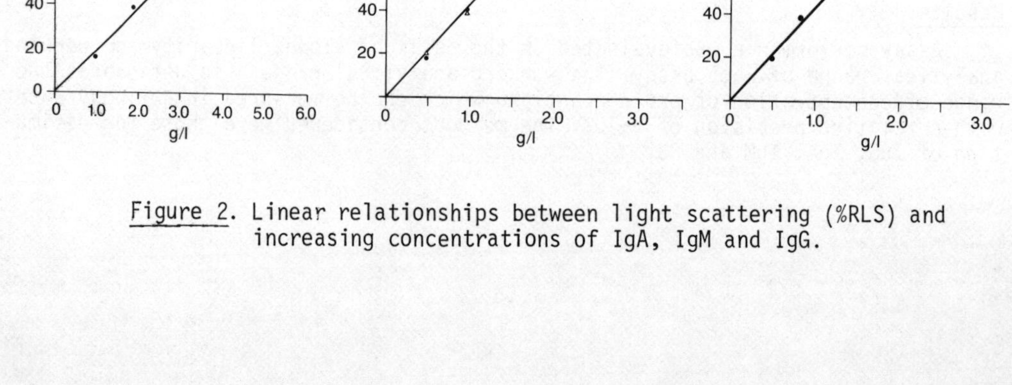

Figure 2. Linear relationships between light scattering (%RLS) and increasing concentrations of IgA, IgM and IgG.

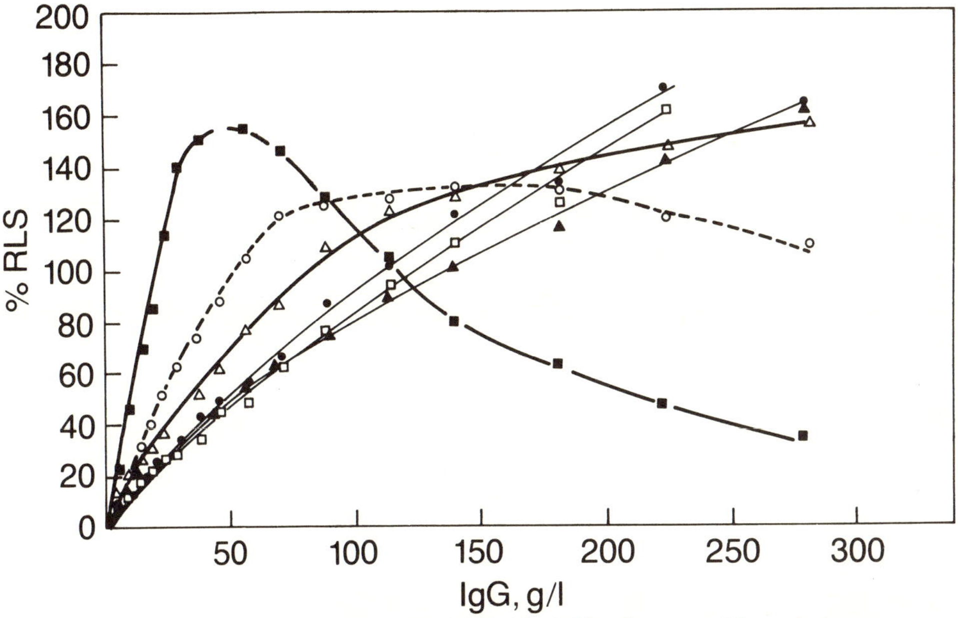

Figure 3. Light scattering (%RLS) following reactions between increasing concentrations of IgG (g/l) and varying dilutions of antibody. The antibody was diluted 1:40 (open square), 1:80 (closed circles), 1:200 (closed triangles), 1:400 (open triangles), 1:800 (open circles) and 1:1600 (closed squares).

For the examination of C3 assay various dilutions of serum and antiserum were used. With only one exception (2μl sample of undiluted serum), all sera were diluted 100-fold before addition to the reaction mixture (Figure 1). In comparison to the prediluted sera, undiluted material resulted in significant curvature to the line relating light scattering to antigen concentration. At high dilution of antiserum, the upper limit of the working analytical range was reduced from 4.0 to 2.75 g/liter as the antiserum dilution was increased from 1:80 to 1:800. Similar studies were done with methods (3,4) developed in this laboratory for assay of IgG, IgA and IgM, all of which gave linear calibration curves (Figure 2). The linear relationship between light scattering and antigen concentration was shown to be a transient phenomenon, even in dilute solution, for if measurements were made after more than 50 minutes linearity was lost.

To evaluate the working analytical range for assay of IgG, IgA and IgM undiluted serum was used to ensure conditions of antigen excess. As shown in Figure 3, the working analytical range for IgG can be increased by using lower dilutions (higher concentrations) of antiserum. Under conditions of antibody excess, as shown also for IgA and IgM on figure 4, the working analytical ranges for IgG, IgA and IgM can be raised to 220, 60 and 32 g/liter, respectively.

To determine whether these observed extended ranges were due to angle of measurement or to the antiserum used, two further comparisons were made. When anti sera from two commercial sources (Hyland and Meloy) were compared in the nephelometer, essentially the same results were obtained for IgG. In a second study, anti sera dilutions recommended for use in clinical situations for the Automated Immunoprecipitation (AIP) System (Table I) were used to assay IgG; in this case scatter

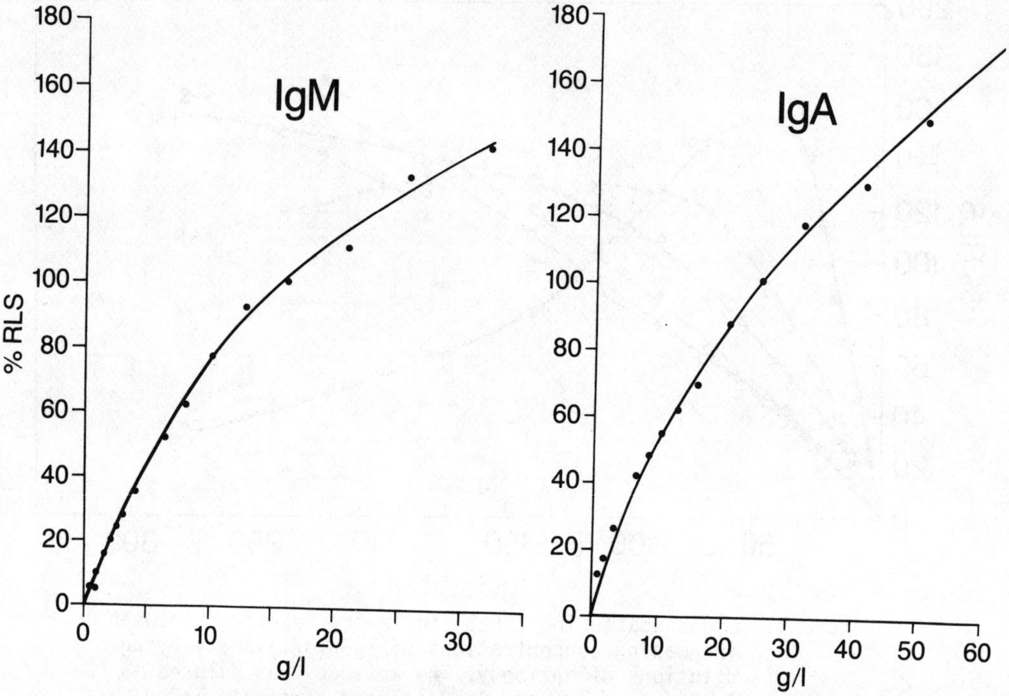

Figure 4. Light scattering (%RLS) under conditions of antibody excess after reaction with increasing amounts of IgM and IgA (g/l).

is measured at 90 instead of 31°. Using antiserum diluted 1:250 IgG could then only be assayed accurately up to a maximum concentration of about 1.70 g/liter.

DISCUSSION

The expected advantage of small angle scattering measurement is to reduce the effect of interference of scattered light associated with macromolecular particles, thereby providing a light scattering signal more closely related to the true particle size and number. We have examined calibration curves for several common assays. The hypothesis is that the relatively limited working analytical range associated with nephelometric assays is caused by use of 90° as the angle of measurement of the light scattering, and that the so called equivalence point is then falsely assigned at a lower antigen concentration than is the actual case. With all assays examined (C3, IgG, IgA, and IgM) the working analytical ranges were significantly greater than those reported for similar methods in which light scattering was measured at 90° (5,6). Since antisera used for the experiments with the IgG assay were from separate commercial sources, we do not believe that the present extended working analytical ranges are due to the titer or avidity of the antiserum. This conclusion is confirmed when antisera from Atlantic Antibodies were used with the Hyland Nephelometer (31°) and the AIP system (90°) for the assay of IgG. It was possible to cover a concentration range of up to 30 g/liter on the Hyland instrument at an antibody dilution of 1:1600 (figure 3) while on the AIP System at a 1:250 dilution of antiserum the concentration range was found to extend only up to 1.7 g/liter.

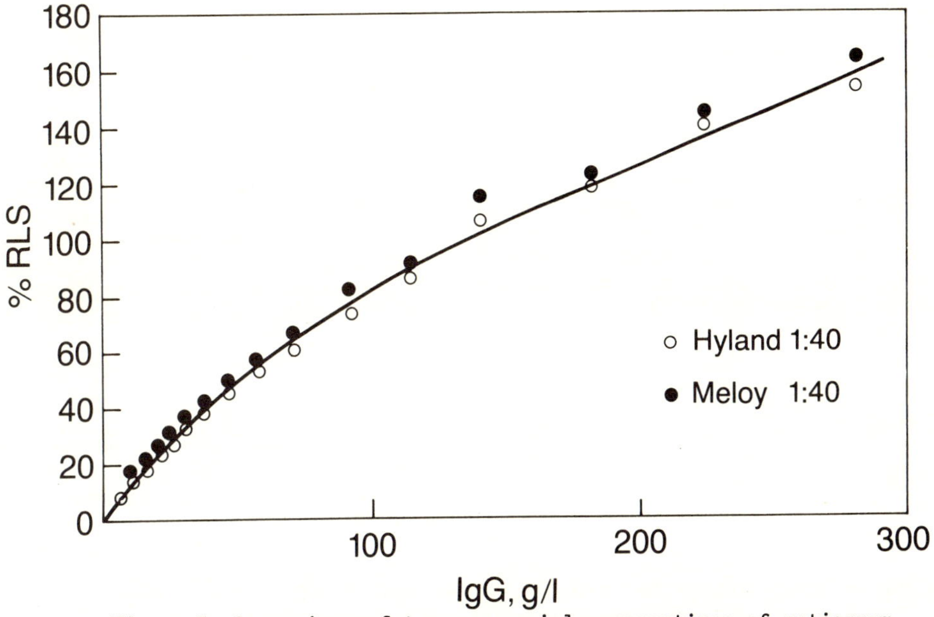

Figure 5. Comparison of two commercial preparations of antiserum (Hyland and Meloy) in the nephelometric assay of IgG. The units used are those defined in other figures.

TABLE I

ANTISERA DILUTIONS FOR THE AIP SYSTEM

PROTEIN	DILUTION *
IgA	1:35
IgG	1:120 (1:250)
IgM	1:40
C3	1:40
C4	1:40
$Alpha_2$macroglobulin	1:40
Haptoglobin	1:100
$Alpha_1$-antitrypsin	1:50
Transferrin	1:120
Albumin	1:50
LDL	1:40
$Alpha_1$-acid glycoprotein	1:60

* These are the dilutions recommended for antisera prepared by Atlantic Antibodies. (Personal Communication; D. Blenkhorn, Atlantic Antibodies, Westbrook, Maine 04092).

Also of interest is the linear relationship between antigen concentration and light scattering intensity. This does not agree with any previous report for immunonephelometric methods, but is in agreement with some kinetic studies performed by the author in 1975 (1). The change in light scattering measured as a function of time for the IgA anti-IgA reaction during the initial phase (<1 min) showed a linear relationship between light scattering and antigen concentration. However, those data and the results of the present study have shown this phenomenon to be transient. It appears that during the initial phase of the reaction in dilute solution a relatively homogeneous particle population exists, both in size and shape, and that only the number of particles varies as a function of antigen concentration. In a more concentrated reaction mixture or after a longer period of reaction, immune complex growth proceeds to the point at which particle heterogeneity becomes significant. Then size, shape and number of particles vary as a function of antigen concentration to give a more complex relationship and significant curvature of the calibration line. This point is illustrated by comparison of the calibration curves for C3 (Figure 1). The use of undiluted calibrators there resulted in marked curvature of the line.

Recently, small volumes of undiluted serum (e.g., 1 to 3 μl) for immunonephelometry have been used to eliminate the need for initial dilution of the sample. As previously described, the curvature seen for this more concentrated system is characteristic of a reaction which has proceeded further toward equilibrium and which in the case of this type of reaction involves precipitation of immune complexes. It is of concern for the analyst to be aware that in some cases (e.g. assay of IgG) formation of large insoluble immune complexes can result in either decreased precision or even erroneous results. In the case of proteins for which an increase in concentration is of clinical significance, the marked curvature will result in a significant loss of sensitivity and decreased precision and accuracy.

In summary there are significant practical advantages to small angle measurement of light scattering for immunonephelometry and the use of dilute solutions provides a more acceptable analytical system for the assay of specific plasma proteins.

REFERENCES

1. Buffone, G.J., Savory, J. and Hermans, J., Evaluation of kinetic light scattering as an approach for the measurement of specific proteins using the centrifugal fast analyzer. II. Theoretical Considerations. Clin.Chem. 21, 1735 (1975)

2. Buffone, G.J., Assay of plasma proteins by immunochemical techniques. Clinical Immunochem. (in press).

3. Buffone, G.J. and Lewis, S.A.,Manual immunochemical nephelometric assays for serum immunoglobulins, IgG, IgA and IgM. Clin.Chem.,(in press)

4. Buffone, G.J. and Lewis, S.A., Effect of analytical factors on immunochemical reference limits for complement component C3 in serum of a reference pediatric population.Clin.Chem.23,994 (1977).

5. Killingsworth, L.M. and Savory, J., Manual Nephelometric methods for immunochemical determination of immunoglobulins, IgG, IgA and IgM in human serum. Clin.Chem.18,335 (1972).

6. Killingsworth, L.M. and Savory, J., Automated immunochemical procedures for measurement of immunoglobulins IgG, IgA and IgM in human serum. Clin.Chem. 17, 1936 (1971).

DISCUSSION

Masson feared interference by coprecipitating agents with light scattering which in fact measures particle size of the antigen/antibody complexes. Even after eliminating the blank due to the presence of lipoprotein, the lypoprotein effect of the antigen/antibody complex is not eliminated. With rheumatoid and Clq, the same problem occurs. Buffone felt that the dilution at which laser nephelometry is performed means that the reading does not respond to the size but to the number of particles. This is why the answers are linear in the range of antigen/antibody ratios used. The protein content of antisera was in the range of 10 ng/ml and, moreover, high affinity antibody was required. De Vreker recalled that all measurements are made in the presence of PEG, in which situation some Igs already transmit turbidity on their own. For this reason, Buffone uses highly diluted prefiltered antisera. Serrera asked whether the coefficient of variation was very different for low and high values. Buffone answers that this coefficient is obviously much higher at very low values. There is no reason why nephelometry should be worse in this respect than any other method,given that the instrumentation as well as the reactants have been optimized. Hobbs claimed that laser nephelometry is much more precise than the Mancini technique when one considers the ordinary laboratory. Even in excellent protein laboratories, the Mancini still gives a precision of only 9-13%. This could be much worse in ordinary laboratories. For this reason laser nephelometry seems an excellent method. Buffone believed that Laser nephelometry is important because it makes absolute measurements available. It appeared from the discussion that random particles, finger prints, etc. greatly can influence results. This means that in spite of all, good laboratory technicians are required but if these conditions are fulfilled the results are very reproducible.

Concluding Comments

Peter H. Wright

Brussels, Belgium

Time alters everything but changes nothing. With the passage of time have come improved Assay techniques with greater sensitivity and specificity. Gone are the days when it was sufficient to assay the protein content of plasma or serum by dropping it into solutions of copper sulphate. In those days, and not so very long ago, it was only necessary to know whether the protein content of plasma was abnormal. If one wished to be sophisticated, one could use a precipitant such as ammonium sulphate to determine whether there was an abnormality of albumin or globulin. Those days are long since gone but the basic problems remain.

As speakers at this symposium have emphasised, attempts are still being made to ensure that the more sophisticated modern methods provide reliable estimates of the nature and quantity of the protein under examination (Hobbs, Engler and Buffone). Adequate sensitivity and specificity are essential for the recognition of proteins characteristic of a clinical condition such as inflammation (Engler); and to establish relative or complete deficiency of specific proteins such as immune globulin (Ballieux). Without reliable diagnostic criteria, rational therapy of deficient states is not possible and new ideas in specific therapy (Masson) cannot be tested. In many apparently auto-immune conditions (Intorp) the underlying causes are still unknown and so rational therapy is still not possible. Many advances have already been made and more must surely come.

Whether by removal of an unwanted toxic protein or by replacement of one that is deficient, treatment is not possible unless the means are available. For removal of toxic substances new methods (e.g. plasmapheresis, hemodialysis, immune suppression, etc.) are being developed. For replacement in the treatment of deficiency states many hormones, vitamins and plasma proteins (De Vreker) are now available, the list being limited only by the present state of man's technical ingenuity.With improvement in techniques will come improvements in our means of diagnosis and in our methods of treatment.

Index